THE LITTLE
TAIJIQUAN MANUAL
FOR BEGINNERS

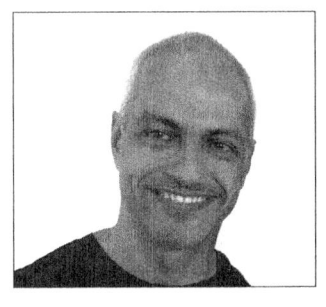

Eduardo Molon started his professional life as an Airline Pilot, following his father's steps.

He started his training in Taijiquan by attending Grandmaster Chen Xiaowang's first seminar in Brazil, in 1998. Chen Xiaowang invited him to stay at his home in Sydney, where Eduardo became an indoor student of Master Chen Yingjun, son of the Grandmaster. He lived for more than two years in Australia, China and Germany to learn Chen family Taijiquan, also receiving intensive training from Jan Silberstorff, under authorization of his Shīfù Chen Yingjun. After 10 years in learning, Eduardo decided to dedicate professionally to Taijiquan, and started teaching in 2008, leaving behind his Aviation career. He organized Master Chen Yingjun's seminars in Brazil for 9 years, directed the World Chen Xiaowang Taijiquan Association in that country, edited the Association's magazine, and trained numerous Instructors certified by it. In 2017, Eduardo was authorized by Master Chen Yingjun to wear his recently created logo.

Eduardo had extensive training in Acupuncture, and ran a private practice in Rio de Janeiro for 8 years.

In 2018, he moved with his family to Ottawa, Canada, where he teaches and from where he broadcasts his online classes.

Website: **https://taijiquan-ottawa.com**
Contact links: **https://eduardomolon.com**
Website in Portuguese: **https://taijiquan.pro.br**
Youtube channel: **https://www.youtube.com/c/chentaijiquan**
Instagram: **@chenyingjun.taijiquan**
Instagram in Portuguese: **@chen.taijiquan**
Facebook: **https://www.facebook.com/chen.taijiquan**
Linkedin: **https://www.linkedin.com/in/eduardomolon**

THE LITTLE TAIJIQUAN MANUAL
FOR BEGINNERS

Eduardo Molon

"Copyright © 2021 Eduardo L. Molon, all rights reserved. No part of this book may be stored in a printed, recorded, electronic or other kind of storage system, nor may it be copied or transmitted by any means, be it printed, recorded, televised, electronic or any other, without previous written consent from the author, except as required by Law."

Design and Desktop Publishing: Walter Mariano
Illustrations: Ian Indiano
Chinese calligraphy: Giankarlo Huback de Almeida

```
Publisher's Cataloging-in-Publishing Data (P-CIP)
```

```
Names: Molon, Eduardo Lucciola
Title: The Little Taijiquan Manual for Beginners
Description: Ottawa, ON - Canada, 2022 | Contents: 1.
Introduction. 2. Basic Knowledge. 3. The Practice of
Taijiquan. 4. Teachings from the Masters.

Identifier: ISBN 9798361312306

Subjects: BISAC:HEALTH & FITNESS / Tai Chi. | SPORTS &
RECREATION / Martial Arts / General.
Classification: DDC 613.7/148
```

Dedication

This modest effort is dedicated to my wife Monica and my children Enzo and Miguel.

Monica, were it not for your unwavering support, I wouldn't have made it to where I am. Thanks to your understanding and acceptance I could pursue my personal goals, while we built a family together.

My sons, this book encloses a message.
It is actually the means I found to record it for you:

There are knowledges that are not academic or intelectual, there is a way of seeing and relating to the universe that is not mechanical nor compartmentalized. There is something sacred and profound that is not religion, there is something silent and subtle that nourishes and pervades everything, and it is possible to connect to it. There is a source of happiness and contentment that does not come from ownership nor contact with others, and it is available to all human beings. There are ways of becoming calm and tranquil and of following the natural order expressed in your mind-body and in your health. Practicing Taijiquan is one way of living these truths. There may be others — I was lucky enough to find this one, and I dreamt of offering it to you.

Safety Recommendations

When starting any physical activity, including Taijiquan, we recommend consulting with your medical doctor to ascertain that you are able to practice it safely. If you have an injury or health condition, consulting with more than one medical doctor, and at least one physical therapist who knows Taijiquan well can be a good idea, since opinions may diverge and can change over time, as it is usual in science.

Don't stop thinking. I have witnessed very intelligent people completely abandon reason simply because a self-proclaimed "master" said a couple of wise sounding sentences. There is no secret mystical force which key, once discovered, will make one strong, skilled and fast. What does exist is a lot of training. Training that is measured in how many hours you put in, not in how many years have passed since you started. Use common sense. Reflect on what you read in this book, and on what you hear from any teacher. Consider whether it is logical, and whether it would apply in the context Taijiquan was created.

Acknowledgements

First and foremost, I'd like to thank my Shīfù, Master Chen Yingjun. When I met him, every time I called him Master, he would say, "I am not a Master yet", for he had many achievements ahead of him. I didn't believe him at that time, because the posture corrections he gave were practically magical. Now, seeing how much he has improved in 21 years, I know he was right — but I am even more positive he has always been a Master to me. He welcomed me in his home, and cared for me as a brother. He did this more than once both in Australia and in China. I would also like to thank his family: his wife, his mother, his sister, his brother, his sister in law and his brother in law, for they all treated me as family, and went above and beyond to make me feel at home, changing their lives and their routines to help me. The feeling of gratitude, in an art like Taijiquan, is very particular, as it grows steadily, even if I don't see my Shīfù as much as I would like to. By practicing every day, as skill improves, so does my gratitude. When you had a real Master to teach you, cultivating your Gongfu is the same as cultivating your gratitude.

My eternal gratitude to my parents, who taught me values that shaped my whole life. Even my Taijiquan practice was shaped by them: I have seen Masters refusing talented students without apparent reason, and when I asked why they did it, they told me "his mind is too unstable" or "he doesn't seem to be a good person". If I was accepted as a student by my Shīfù, it was thanks to how my parents raised me.

I am very thankful to Grandmaster Chen Xiaowang. Thanks to his generosity in traveling around the world to teach, I found real Taijiquan, and thanks to his intervention I found my Shīfù. I also want to thank Master Jan Silberstorff, to whom Taijiquan's development in Brazil, and my own, are deeply indebted.

I extend my gratitude to Acacio Suzuki Sensei, my Master in Acupuncture. Thanks to his teachings I could have a brief insight of how and where Acupuncture and Taijiquan meet. I thank my brother Giankarlo Huback for the beautiful Chinese calligraphy in this book and for his unfailing companionship and wise advice along my life; my dear friend Daniel Luz for the etymology of the Chinese characters found here and for always sharing with me everything that was dear to him; my good friends Liana, Beto and Lara, and Ralf Anlauf, for welcoming me in their homes; and all my friends in Taijiquan practice, specially Mario Gusmão, Bob Melo, Jucival, Flávio Octaviani, Robson, Flávio Pessoa, Luciano and Jader. I thank all my students, present and past, as they always challenged me to practice more so I could teach them better, which had me keep drinking directly from the source, where the water is clearer.

I thank very specially this book's Designer, Walter Mariano. This book was first imagined by him, and it wouldn't exist hadn't he pushed me to write it. Finally I thank Ian Indiano for his beautiful drawings and his effort in translating my words into images.

Words from Master Chen Yingjun

Eduardo is a very good student and friend of mine. I know his family very well, from my visits to Rio de Janeiro, when I taught the seminars he organized for me for many years. He also knows my family very well.

Eduardo started learning from me in 2001. He made long and hard trips from Rio to Sydney and to China, to have intensive training with me in private lessons. His longest stay was about one and a half years. Not only did he make those trips for studying with me, he has been training according to my way for a very long time, and very diligently. He has a very good level of understanding in the art.

I hope that, with this book, he will help many beginners in the start of their learning in Taijiquan.

Chen Yingjun

Preface to the English edition

The original, Portuguese version of this book was finished in 2017. This translation to English is now offered as I have since moved to Canada, and have been building my Master's school in Ottawa.

As the English language might extend the reach of my humble efforts to a wider audience than Portuguese, I must remind the reader that all merit in this book is my Shīfù's, and all shortcomings are mine.

Thanks to my Shīfù's support and teachings, my understanding of Taijiquan has changed since I wrote this text, as it is supposed to, and I plan to write a second volume reflecting those changes. I chose to translate the original text to English without any updating, because it is meant for beginners. The explanations herein are needed as stepping stones, so they can come to understand the next volume.

Table of Contents

INTRODUCTION

13 **Target audience, and what to expect from this book**
How this book is organized
14 **Short autobiographical account**
16 **Not everything that is called Taijiquan, is really Taijiquan**
17 **About didactic material**

BASIC KNOWLEDGE

20 **Context and History**
22 **Yin and Yang**
Applications for the human body
24 **Qi or Vital Energy**
Does Qi exist, or not?
27 **Acupuncture Channels**
35 **A complete system**
A method for generating power
Applications training
Aerobic training
Stretching
Qigong exercises
Concentration and meditation
Simplifications and modern didactics
How to practice Taijiquan
More on accessory exercises

TAIJIQUAN PRACTICE

- 39 **Values**
  - Loyalty
  - Propriety
  - Dedication
  - Honesty
  - Integrity
  - How to find a good teacher
  - What is Gongfu (or Kungfu)
- 44 **Technique, Technology and Principles**
  - Principles
- 46 **Didactics**
  - Didactics, Principles, and Method
  - Common questions
- 52 **Strength, Qi, Jin, and Qigong**
  - Qigong or Chi Kung
  - Taoist Alchemy
  - Taijiquan Masters, and Tuishou
- 60 **Fengshui**
- 64 **Body positioning**
  - Head
  - Shoulders and arms
  - Chest
  - Spine
  - Hips
  - Knees
  - Feet
- 71 **Zhanzhuang**
- 83 **Chansigong**
  - Yin and Yang in motion
  - Didactics of Silk Reeling
  - Remarks on common mistakes
  - Moving on
- 105 **Forms**

MASTERS' TEACHINGS

- 120 **Listen carefully**
- 121 **Living teachings**
- 122 **It's easier to teach a child**
- 123 **Do only one thing**
- 124 **Naturalness**
- 126 **The teacher follows first**
- 127 **You can't teach a skill**
- 128 **Relaxation and posture**
- 129 **The cause of strengthening**
- 130 **Breathing**
- 131 **With Qi only**
- 132 **Best time for practice**
- 133 **It is necessary to change**
- 134 **Leave your neck out of it**
- 135 **Do not pull your knees out**
- 136 **Feet position**
- 137 **Teacher's skill**
- 138 **Focus**
- 139 **Trying to copy what you can't do**
- 140 **Posture height**
- 141 **First, Qi returns to Dantian**
- 142 **Don't look for feelings**
- 143 **Pain**
- 144 **Raise your average**
- 145 **Light arms**
- 146 **Speed of practice**
- 150 **Five Levels of Gongfu**
  - Introduction
  - The first level of Gongfu
  - The second level of Gongfu
  - The third level of Gongfu
  - The fourth level of Gongfu
  - The fifth level of Gongfu

Introduction

Target audience, and what to expect from this book

There are several kinds of books on Taijiquan. Usually, a Master writes a book about the art once they reach a high skill level. Masters' books commonly show movement sequences, with photos featuring the author in strong and stable postures, meant to guide and inspire students. They may also contain historical accounts and explanations of the principles and the profound theory underlying the art. None of these are to be found in this book. This is a book written by a teacher, and it will not describe movement sequences or theory at a deep philosophical level.

This book is a manual for interpreting and applying instructions that Masters impart. When we start learning Taijiquan, we are faced with a completely new field of knowledge. We are re-introduced to our body and its nature, seen from the perspective of a culture and a way of thinking that are very different from the Western ones. This causes Taijiquan's learning curve to be very steep at the beginning. A lot of time, and a lot of effort, is wasted struggling to overcome our own difficulty in communicating with someone who belongs to another culture - even if they speak a common language - and who possesses completely different and rather unique body and movement knowledge. This book is an attempt in making the learning curve smoother for the beginner, and in avoiding unnecessary efforts in the wrong direction, so the student's energy and time can be employed in the most rewarding fashion.

HOW THIS BOOK IS ORGANIZED

After going through some basic knowledge, the book is organized following the ideal sequence in a typical class: Zhanzhuang (Standing Meditation), Chansigong (Silk Reeling Qigong), and Forms (the sequences of Taijiquan movements). The chapter on the Masters' teachings follows a compatible order, that is, it begins and ends at the same points where the chapter on practice begins and ends - except for the text on the Five Levels of Gongfu, which is almost a separate book in itself.

Short autobiographical account

It is necessary to recount a little about my personal story, so the reader, having known of it, can share my point of view at least in part.

I became interested in Taijiquan by pure chance, when I saw a group practicing in a public square in Rio de Janeiro, where I lived, in 1989. The internet didn't exist at the time, and even fax machines weren't widespread. It was not possible to watch a Taijiquan Master performing on YouTube - what you saw at the nearest public square was all that was available. I started practicing with that group, and after 8 years in training, my left knee was in such serious trouble that I couldn't even go down stairs. I was injured during practice, around the third or fourth year. I was so very stubborn that I continued pushing forward, when any measure of common sense would have made me stop, but I thought I was persevering. The "teacher" said my body was changing, and if I pushed through, the pain would just go away. The injury became so severe that three different Orthopaedic Medical Doctors recommended surgery, and two Physiotherapists said that they saw no way for recovery without it. But I didn't want to stop practicing, and knee surgery at the age of 28 didn't seem like a good bet. It is necessary to strongly emphasize that nowadays I would not call what I practiced then by the name of Taijiquan. What I practiced at the start of the 90's caused a knee injury, and Taijiquan in contrast should be good for your health, especially for your joint health. All of the theory I was taught was correct - but the practical instructions on how to align and move the body were completely wrong. A few of my friends in that group were also seriously injured. I eventually left that group, looked for alternative exercises, but I kept the postural errors with me, because I had trained my body that way, and continued suffering with my injured knee, in chronic pain.

Grandmaster Chen Xiaowang went to Brazil for the first time in 1998. He is the heir of the 19th generation of the Chen family, which created Taijiquan in the 17th century. Many of the founder's descendants still live in the same village as their ancestor, Chenjiagou, where they run a Taijiquan school. I happened to receive a brochure of his seminar, and decided to enrol. I was lucky enough in being able to book several private lessons with him. On the first practice day, Chen Xiaowang offered a demonstration. Thirty or forty people were sitting on folding chairs, staring at him, in a gym. When he started, his explosive power was so intense that the thirty chairs were moved a foot backwards, pushed by the people sitting on them, amazed. The contrast with what I knew was so stark that I immediately understood I had never even seen Taijiquan before, let alone practice it. Contrast during class was identical. As soon as the

Grandmaster corrected my posture, my knee pain disappeared. I couldn't believe it. Not just that: the difficulty going down the stairs, which had been with me for a couple of years, was completely gone. The improvement was not permanent, and some hours later, as soon as my body resumed its usual posture, the problems were back. But in all private lessons the same effect repeated[1].

I practiced alone until the following year, when Chen Xiaowang went to Brazil a second time. When I had my first private lesson, the effect of his posture corrections continued to surprise and impress me, but finding out that I needed adjustments to my posture as large and deep as the year before was very disappointing. I naively thought I would be more successful if I practiced for yet another year, and planned measuring my improvement in the next meeting with Chen Xiaowang. He returned again in the year 2000, and again I was frustrated by my lack of progress: large adjustments, their impressive effects, and the feeling of not having improved, even though I had been practicing diligently. It became clear my improvement pace would not be satisfactory if I met him only once a year. I had just read that Chen Xiaowang had a son living in Australia, who also taught Taijiquan. During one of the breaks in a private lesson, I asked him if he thought traveling to Sydney on my vacations and learning from his son, Chen Yingjun, would be a good idea. Right there my fate was changed: the Grandmaster replied, "you live with me". He offered me to stay at his house, and to arrange with his son for my stay and my classes in Australia.

That's how I became an indoor student of Chen Yingjun.

---

[1] This is my personal history, and not a treatment suggestion. If you have a health condition like this, please see your doctor first.

Not everything that is called Taijiquan, is really Taijiquan

Directing the reader's attention to a specific part of my personal story is imperative: between 1989 and 1998, I practiced something that was sold to me as Taijiquan, but did not nearly deserve the name.

Copying the outward appearance of Taijiquan is not too difficult for someone with only moderate movement experience, as its movements are almost always performed at a slow pace. Someone who practiced martial arts before can learn the forms fairly quickly, and can demonstrate them with great aesthetic appeal, if they are flexible enough and show low postures. Understanding what one is doing is a completely different matter. A Chen family Taijiquan Master, on the other hand, starts training when 4 or 5 years old. When high school ends, their parents start their professional training regimen, and they dedicate exclusively to it, from 17 or 18 years old to about 40. After about twenty years under high level instruction in full time training, a Chen descendant will be a Master, that is, they will have mastered their ancestors' art. Be it clear there is an insurmountable abyss between the first and the second cases above.

It can be said Taijiquan is a Martial Art, as its creator's descendants firmly assert. It can be said it is a health practice, a philosophy for life, or a means to follow a spiritual path. Taijiquan is so flexible and adaptable it can be reframed according to how each person uses it. But there are minimal technical and pragmatic requirements for calling something Taijiquan. From a technical point of view, it is necessary that the body posture constantly aims to obey the Three External Harmonies, and that each and every movement aims to be executed according to Silk Reeling principles. I am forced to write "aims to", because these are very demanding requirements, and it takes an actual Master to fulfill them all the time. From a practical point of view, it is quite simple: something called Taijiquan should, at the very least, be good for your joints and general health. Something bringing on injuries and joint problems cannot be called Taijiquan.

This short account is intended as an alert for the reader, so they constantly assess their practice and their sources of instruction. Do not abandon logic and common sense. It is all too usual, in many different types of sports, to witness this.

About didactic material

All Taijiquan teaching material, including this book, is meant for learning support only. This refers to books, videos, and audio recordings. Learning Taijiquan without direct, in person lessons with a very good teacher is impossible; and it is essential, at least once every few years, to attend a Master's seminar. Your teacher must correct your body posture with their own hands. They have to adjust your hip position, your spine's shape, and your limbs' alignments. A Master is like a compass, so you can be sure of where you are going. Neither of these two sources can be replaced.

It is worth remembering every teacher can only teach according to their level. Everything described in this book is correct for my level of training in 2017, when I wrote the manuscript. I am sure some years later I will read this Manual's manuscript and I will find numerous gaps. There is no remedy for it, unless we were talking about a Master like Chen Xiaowang, Chen Fake, or a Chen ancestor.

Taijiquan is the very image of Dao, reflected by human movement. The first verse of the Daodejing says:

What one can say of Dao, is not the real Dao.

This means when one tries to describe the Indescribable with words, one cannot do it. The same applies to Taijiquan. As it is Dao reflected by the human body, every time you try to explain it, every time you try to put in words what the body movement should be like when you are following the laws of Yin and Yang, you are simplifying it. Any description of Taijiquan is bound to be limited.

One could thus say everything you read in this book is "wrong". That would be a bit of an exaggeration as, in order to start practicing, we need explanations and guidance. That is - except if you were born in the Chen family, you are the son of a Master, you were raised the old fashioned way and began practicing as a child, when your mind was clear of prejudice. This book is therefore constrained to a specific context. After a few years practicing, depending on how many hours a day you put in, I hope you will find this book too limited. It will have then fulfilled its purpose.

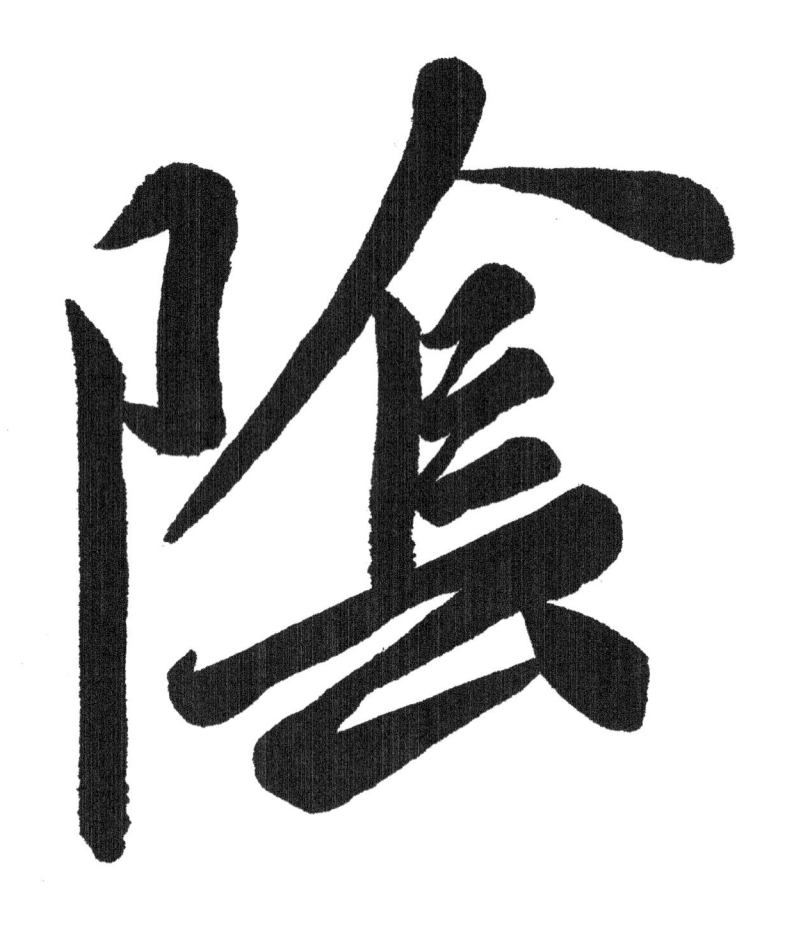

Yīn (陰): on the left, mountain; on the right, jīn 今, now, over yūn 云, saying (classical), clouds.
Yáng (陽): on the left, mountain; on the right, dàn 旦, dawn, morning, over 勿 wù, flags waving on the wind, used to signal troop movement during battles, denial, no.

The ideograms must be analyzed together. They are the two sides of a mountain: the image of "now" ("to grab three") is contrasted with "sunrise", when the sun is seen above the horizon,

陽

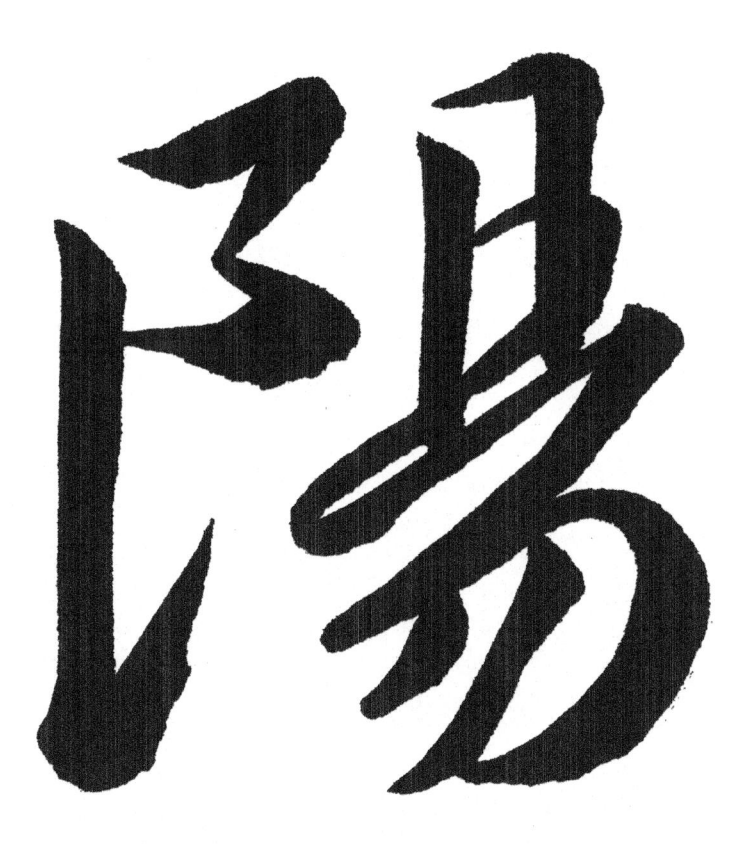

an image of a trajectory, of flowing time; in the lower part at the right, in Yīn we have the obscurity of clouds on a mountain's side; in Yáng we have flags clearly signalling movement that can and that cannot be undertaken. Yīn is the present time and the undefined path of clouds going about a mountain's side, Yáng is the sunny side of flowing time and clear and lively movement.

Basic Knowledge

Context and History

The martial art now bearing the name Taijiquan was systematized by Chen Wangting (1600-1680), a local military commander in Wen District (Wenxian), central China, in the 19th century. Chen Wangting did not create Taijiquan out of nowhere. His ancestors were already martial artists, even before migrating to Henan province. Before retiring in 1644, due to the fall of the Ming dynasty, to which he was loyal, Chen Wangting learned various techniques and martial styles and was influenced by these and other body techniques found in China, such as Duna and Daoyin. The current outward aspect of Chen family Taijiquan is not exactly the same as it was 380 years ago: both appearance and content have been refined over generations, from Chen Wangting's 9th generation to the present 19th generation, which patriarch is Grandmaster Chen Xiaowang. Chen Xiaowang's sons and nephews are the 20th generation Masters in the Chen family.

French historians Thomas Dufresne and Jacques Nguyen, supported, among others, by the field research of famous Chinese historian Tang Hao (1897-1959), propose the hypothesis that the style created by Chen Wangting descends from martial styles of Generals Yu Dayou (1503-1579) and Qi Jiguang (1528-1588). General Qi Jiguang was sent to save the situation in a battle against the Wokou in the 16th century, where many others had failed. The famous General was successful in battle and his martial style gained great prestige. Qi Jiguang authored the Jixiao Xinshu, a treatise containing 32 illustrated techniques and a synthesis of 16 martial styles from late Ming dynasty. The martial treatises of Qi Jiguang and Yu Dayou have several techniques in common, and it is thought that Yu Dayou taught his staff style to Qi Jiguang. They likely practiced at least similar martial styles. The name of twenty nine of the thirty two techniques described by Qi Jiguang are found among the ancient techniques of Taijiquan. It is noteworthy that although nowadays knowledge of names and descriptions of techniques is open, knowing the style in depth was necessary to gain such access at that time. The martial art created by Chen Wangting, Taijiquan, is however unique in many ways, not found in any of its predecessors, which bears witness to his genius. He founded a unique style, improved upon by successive generations of descendants.

One other source of influence was probably important for creating Taijiquan, in addition to Qi Jiguang: the Huang Ting Jing, or Yellow Courtyard Classic, a book written in the 3rd or 4th century by Daoist nun Wei Huacun. This book may have been the main source of energy circulation techniques found in Taijiquan.

Chen Wangting was an experienced battlefield warrior. Picture a medieval war: hundreds of spearmen, thousands of foot soldiers wielding broadswords, a dozen officers on horseback armed with halberds, perhaps a detachment of archers. Two armies like this meeting at an open field. There is no fighting in such a setup, there is only killing. Chen Wangting was molded by this experience and he trained his descendants for this kind of environment. The Chen family, which had been on the loyalist side at the fall of Ming dynasty, was out of official military milieu for a few generations, but eventually returned. Chen Changxing, 14th generation, was a commercial caravan security officer: he led the security of caravans carrying goods in mainland China, at a time when public policing was practically non-existent. He could be attacked anytime by an unknown number of brigands, with any existing weapons. The 15th generation Chen family Masters defended their village, leading somewhere between 1,000 and 2,000 men, against a Taiping contingent ten times that size, for long enough to allow the region to be evacuated.

Chen Wangting was a Warlord. He belonged to a clan of warriors, and was raised to follow the path of arms. By systematizing his knowledge into Taijiquan, he did so to faithfully pass it on to future generations of his family. He did not create a foot soldier quick training program, rather a system for training his descendants, from childhood, to be professional military officers. An infantry recruit is an expendable piece in a Middle Age battle, and was given brief training to become useful in a few months. A martial clan warrior began training at the age of 5 or 6, on a full-time basis, and was ready for war in his early thirties. This is the knowledge that is preserved in Taijiquan.

Yin and Yang

At a time when available technology was limited, some people in China cultivated a very special way of observing nature. As they looked outward - at natural phenomena around them, such as the passing of seasons, the revolving of stars in the sky, and other natural cycles - they simultaneously looked inward. Through self-observation and meditation, those we now call sages were able to distinguish correspondences between macrocosm and microcosm, between nature and man.

They found all phenomena then observable could be described by means of a dichotomy: two interacting, opposing principles. These principles were called Yin and Yang. Originally, the character for Yin meant the northern face of a mountain, and the one for Yang meant the southern face. The sun is never at the zenith in the northern hemisphere, above the Tropic of Cancer - not even at midday. This means the northern face, or Yin side of a mountain, never gets the same amount of sunlight as the southern face, or Yang side. There is therefore less activity on the Yin face, less butterflies, less birds, more moisture and moss, less light. There is more activity on the Yang face: more movement, more exuberance and warmth. The names Yin and Yang in this context have no positive or negative connotations, specially no moral connotation of good or evil. The sages and meditators could then understand certain natural laws to which all manifestations obey, how these two principles unfold, how they interact and manifest.

The most economic formulation of these natural laws is illustrated in the Taiji Tu, the diagram showing Yin and Yang interacting. What does the diagram mean? The four main characteristics governing all phenomena are condensed in a single drawing:

- In any situation or event, *two interacting, opposing principles* can be found.
- These principles *are complementary*, that is, one does not exist without the other, it is not possible to isolate them.
- The two principles *alternate in time*, increasing and decreasing one after the other.
- They *generate each other*, that is, when one of them reaches its apex, the opposing principle's seed arises inside it.

Water show qualities of Yin: deep, heavy, slow, dark, dense, cold; and fire show qualities of Yang: rising, light, fast, clear, rarefied, hot. It is of course not possible to describe everything in detail using the two principles at this level of simplification. One is forced to unfold Yin and

Yang into its four appearances: Young Yin, Mature Yin, Young Yang, and Mature Yang, which follow each other in this very order. If we further increase our resolution, we get the Eight Trigrams, which are the basis for the Yi Jing (or I Ching), an ancient Chinese civilization classic sometimes used as an oracle, which is actually a description of the relationship between the two natural principles and their transformations.

APPLICATIONS FOR THE HUMAN BODY

The human body is subject to the same natural laws as any other phenomenon or part of nature. In the same way as in day and night, and in the seasons of the year and their cycle, one can see the manifestation of Yin and Yang in the human body.

The anatomical position used in Chinese Medicine is slightly different from that in Bio-Medicine. The subject is standing with arms up, toes pointing outwards, and palms facing forward. This is the appropriate position for describing the areas under stronger influence of Yin or Yang:

- The top (from the waist up) is Yang, and the bottom (from the waist down) is Yin.
- The dorsal side is Yang, and the ventral side is Yin.
- The centre is more Yin, and the periphery is more Yang.
- The inside of the body is more Yin, and its outside is more Yang.

Qi or Vital Energy

Master Chen Yingjun was once asked during a seminar, "What is Qi, this energy that people talk about so much? Where does it come from? From the Cosmos, from the Universe?" Unable to hide his surprise, he replied, as if the student had asked the most obvious question of all: "it's the energy in the food you eat". No one practicing Taijiquan in the Chenjiagou village is at all concerned with esotericism, rather with finding out what works and what doesn't in the realm of concrete application.

What western culture calls Energy and Chinese culture calls Qi is for those raised in that culture a very real and concrete thing. Saying Qi moves from the centre of the body to one's hands is as concrete as saying there's friction when a chair rubs while being dragged across the floor. This is a perfect analogy by the way. When you enter high school and start studying Physics, you learn how to calculate the friction force between the ground and an object dragged on it. Friction is part of your everyday sensory experience: you feel it every time you drag a chair you're sitting on. Friction, however, doesn't actually exist. Try asking a Physicist if there is a force in nature called friction, and they will tell you that the friction you experience every day is actually electromagnetism: on the outside of the atoms that make up matter are electrons, which have a negative charge. Negative charges repel each other, and as the surfaces are irregular rather than flat as they appear to the naked eye, irregularities repel each other in the horizontal direction, making movement difficult. Any Physicist will tell you there are only four forces in nature: electromagnetism, gravity, strong, and weak (the latter two, within atoms only). You're not wrong, however, when talking about friction. Engineers use this concept to design from matchsticks to airplanes. Friction is a useful and necessary abstraction, as it would be impossible to design planes, cars or rockets, calculating the repulsion forces between every pair of electrons.

DOES QI EXIST OR NOT?
This is a moot point. The question doesn't even make sense, it's the same as asking whether friction exists or not. This is not to say it is acceptable to mystify the concept and believe in a semi-ethereal substance that permeates the entire Cosmos. What matters to us is that you can train yourself to feel and use what Chinese culture calls Qi, in order to align your posture, guide movement and optimize power transmission inside your body.

Take another example: you truly believe that there is such a thing as muscle power. If you are lifting weights, an instructor might say, "engage your lats," and you wouldn't find it strange, as the feeling of contracting a muscle is something all too familiar, and present in your everyday life, but there is no such thing as muscle power for a Physicist. What is actually involved in shortening a muscle, and which causes a limb to move, are electromagnetic bonds between the atoms in the myofibrils that make up your muscles. It just doesn't make sense for a weightlifting instructor to say, "change the molecular bonds of your muscle fibres in such a way." That would be useless, as this instruction is not actionable because the problem of which atomic bonds to change is intractable from this point of view. You and the instructor choose to use a mutually agreed upon abstraction that you both know as muscle engagement. Chinese culture offers you a different abstraction for dealing with the problem of integral body movement. It is called Qi. It is simply a historical anecdote that the Chinese Qi character was translated as energy. This abstraction is commonplace for anyone raised in Chinese culture, and is nothing new for a Taijiquan beginner in China. If you want to learn to move the body holistically and in a coordinated way as prescribed by Taijiquan, your teacher needs to use this abstraction to explain the movement, as well as several other culture-specific concepts. If they try to use instructions like "engage that muscle", the problem of how to move the body in the special way Taijiquan prescribes becomes intractable, and they won't be able to teach you.

Chen Xiaowang likes to draw analogies to driving cars when he first explains the basics of practice. I would say: you cannot teach someone to drive by telling the learner which muscles to use. If you are a driving instructor and you tell a student learning how to drive a stick-shift car, "contract the right quadriceps with your foot on the clutch pedal", then "contract the right biceps while holding the gear lever" to shift gears, they won't understand a thing. What you do in real life is tell them to press the clutch pedal and engage the second gear.

We can also draw a software analogy. Imagine you are trying to program a computer. In the 1980s, there were still machine language manuals in specialist bookstores. You could buy such a manual, and learn how to directly program an 8088 processor. An 80's microprocessor didn't know how multiply: you had to write a subroutine in which you instructed the processor to do several additions, only then it would be able to multiply one integer by another. This is called low-level programming, and machine language is a low-level programming language. Below this level are the transistors - any microprocessor is a huge web of transistors that open or close, allowing or stopping the flow of electric current and performing the operations we know. Some computer games from that decade were written in low-level language for faster execution. It would not be possible to write a computer game, not even in the 80s, describing which transistors should open and which should close, on every infinitesimal part of a second - it would be just too complicated. The processing power of computers grew over time, programs became much more complex, and games became way more realistic. Today they are programs so big and complex that it would be impossible to write them using direct instructions for the microprocessor. New programming languages were created to allow ever broader abstractions: they are the high-level languages. In this analogy, the molecules in your muscles which changing bonds shorten and extend muscle fibres are the transistors in microprocessors. Dealing with them is not the programmer's job, it's the electronic engineer's. If you're still exercising using "engage that muscle" instructions, you're like a programmer still using a low-level programming language to command your body, which is capable of way more and better than that. It's time to upgrade your operating system, and start using a high-level programming language, with much broader and more powerful abstractions: the circulation of vital energy, Qi.

It is important to remember the interpretation proposed above is not nearly exhaustive. It only applies to body movement, and is insufficient for other contexts outside our scope, like Acupuncture. However, the same line of thought can be applied to weave similar analogies. The concept of Qi is broader, deeper, and more important than what I explained above. Mine was a discussion restricted to the context of the Taijiquan movement at a basic level. It is helpful in making Qi a more palatable concept for the beginner, but it is far from being complete even in this restricted context. Qi is a prevalent concept in Chinese culture, and is applied to physiological, mental, and natural processes that are beyond the scope of this book.

For now, we can say Qi circulation, in the context of movement, is a measure of the Taijiquan students's skill in transmitting spiral power through their body.

Acupuncture Channels

Meridian is a misnomer for the Qi pathways described by Acupuncture. They are in fact called Channels, in the same sense as an irrigation channel, as that is what they do: they irrigate the body with Qi, like arteries irrigate the body with blood. There is no "proof" Acupuncture channels "exist", to this day. However, proving and existing in this context makes as little sense as I earlier explained when discussing whether Qi exists, for what matters to us is that the concept works and is very useful. An Acupuncture channel is sometimes represented on a map with a line. We therefore tend to think Qi circulates in the body along these imaginary lines, which in reality is a reductionist outlook. Believing blood circulates in the body only in main arteries would be an equivalent reduction. Every tissue in the body, every living part of the body, has energy circulating through it, and the channels we remember when we talk about Acupuncture are just the main ones. The main channels have names relating to the internal organs where they originate, and also have older names indicating the "energy level" between the Yin and Yang extremes where they sit. For example: Shou Taiyang and Zu Taiyang are the Yang-most main channels in the body, respectively in the hand and foot. If we refer only to the Taiyang channel, we are talking about the Grand Taiyang Channel, which runs from top to bottom in the body, from hand to foot. In a more complete Acupuncture atlas, you can find the tendon-muscle channel pathways, which bear the same names as the main channels. For example: tendon-muscle Bladder channel, etc. These channels are on the paths of the muscle groups around and following the main energy channels' paths. Knowledge of the tendon-muscle channels is useful, although not essential, for Taijiquan students. See the Shou Taiyang and the Zu Taiyang, and then check out their tendon-muscle channels, and you will know one of the paths by which the hand and foot (and thus the whole body) are connected.

As practice progresses, it is possible to feel that in a good posture, the internal alignments of the muscles consistently follow the paths of the tendon-muscle channels of the Great Channels mapped by Acupuncture, forming actual mechanical connections.

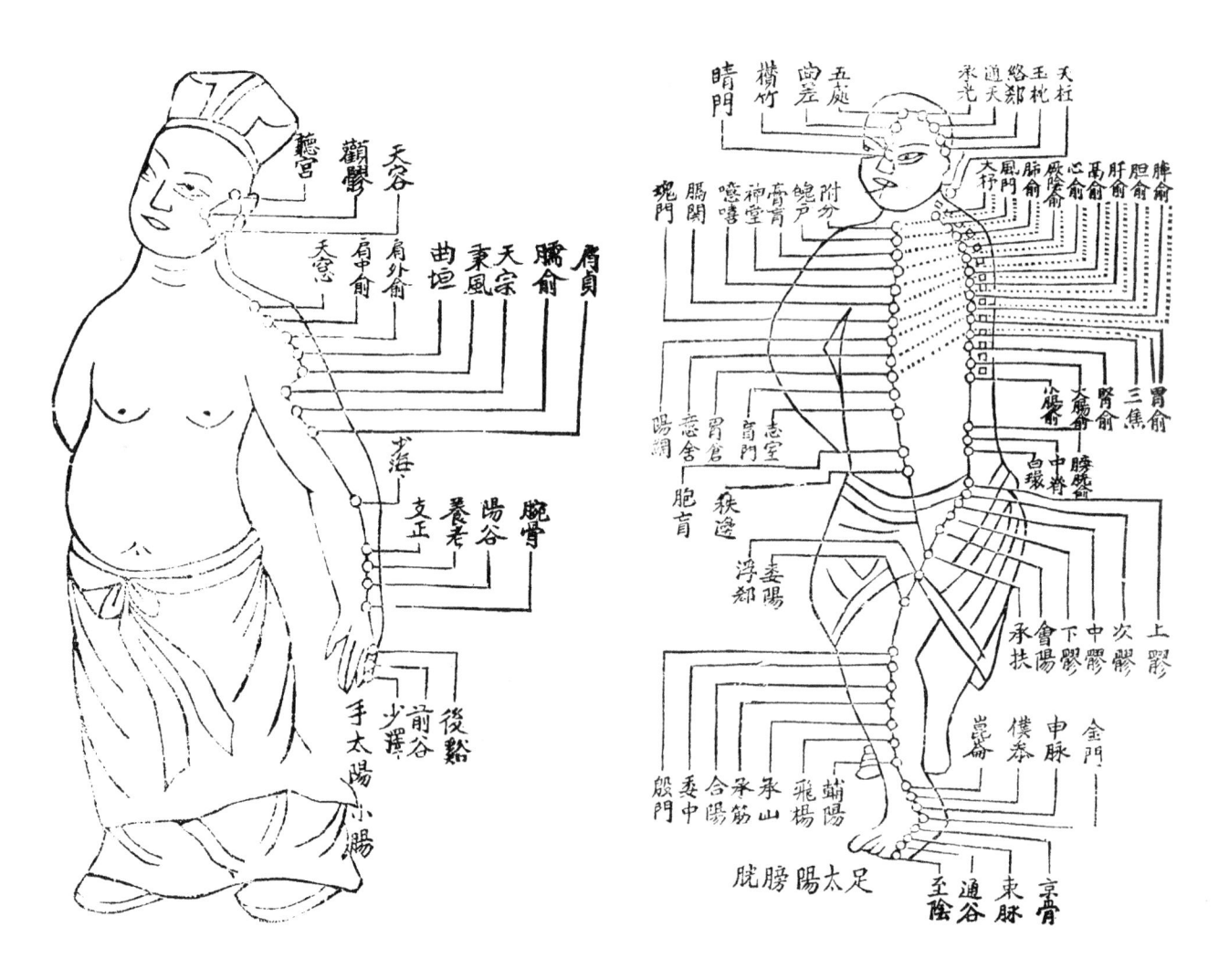

Shou Taiyang [2.4.1]

Zu Taiyang [2.4.2]

THE LITTLE TAIJIQUAN MANUAL FOR BEGINNERS

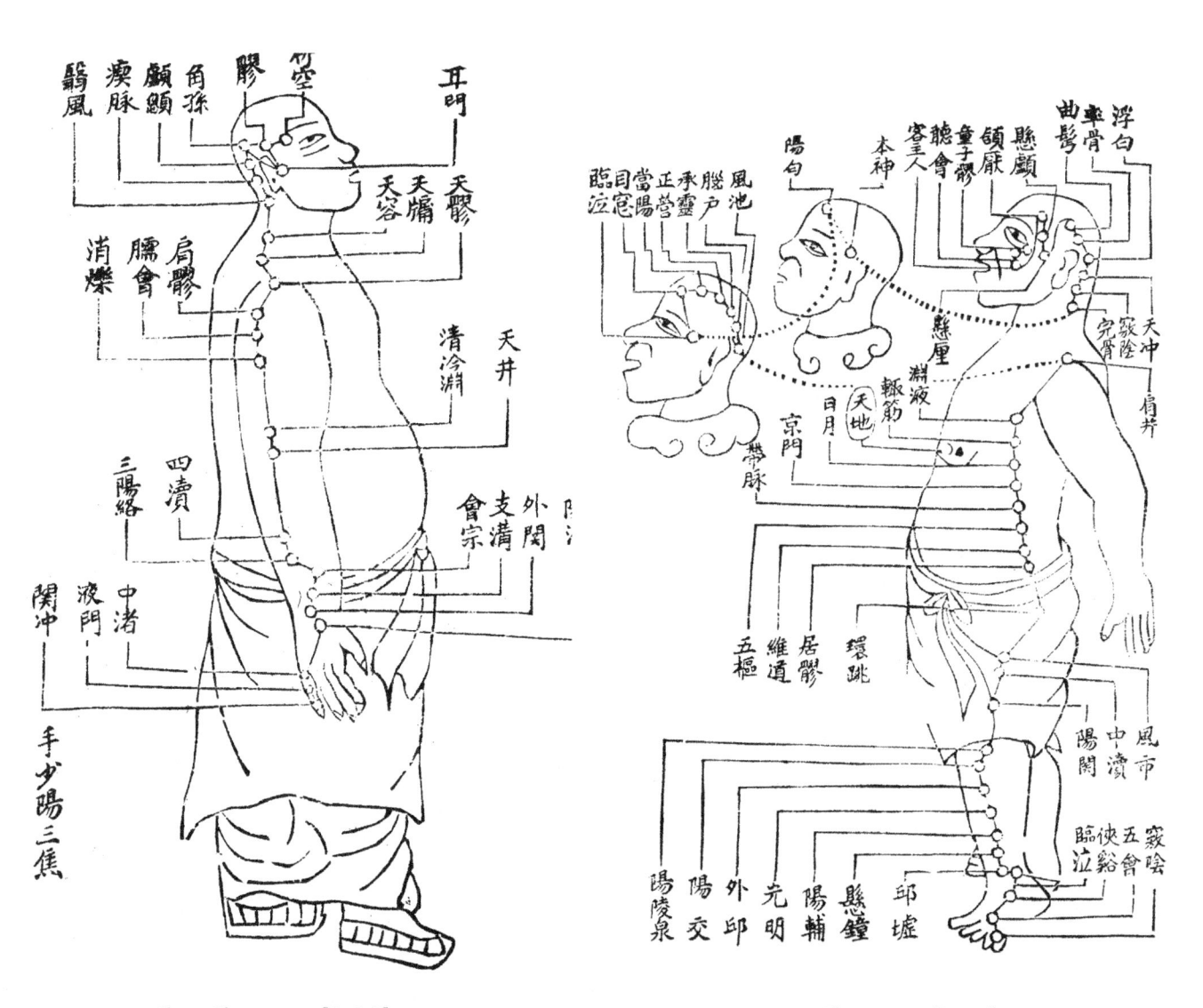

Shou Shaoyang [2.4.3]

Zu Shaoyang [2.4.4]

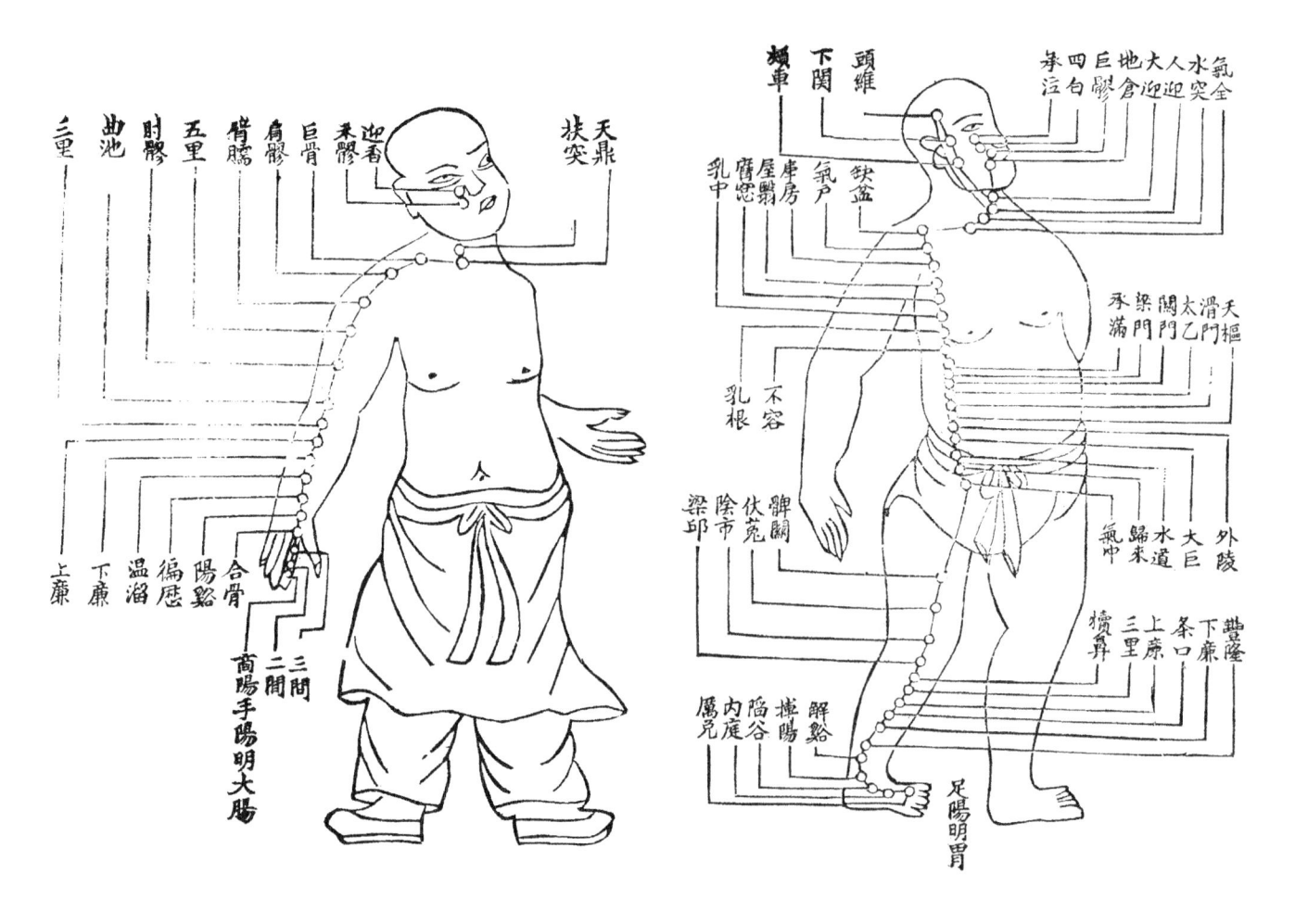

Shou Yangming [2.4.5]

Zu Yangming [2.4.6]

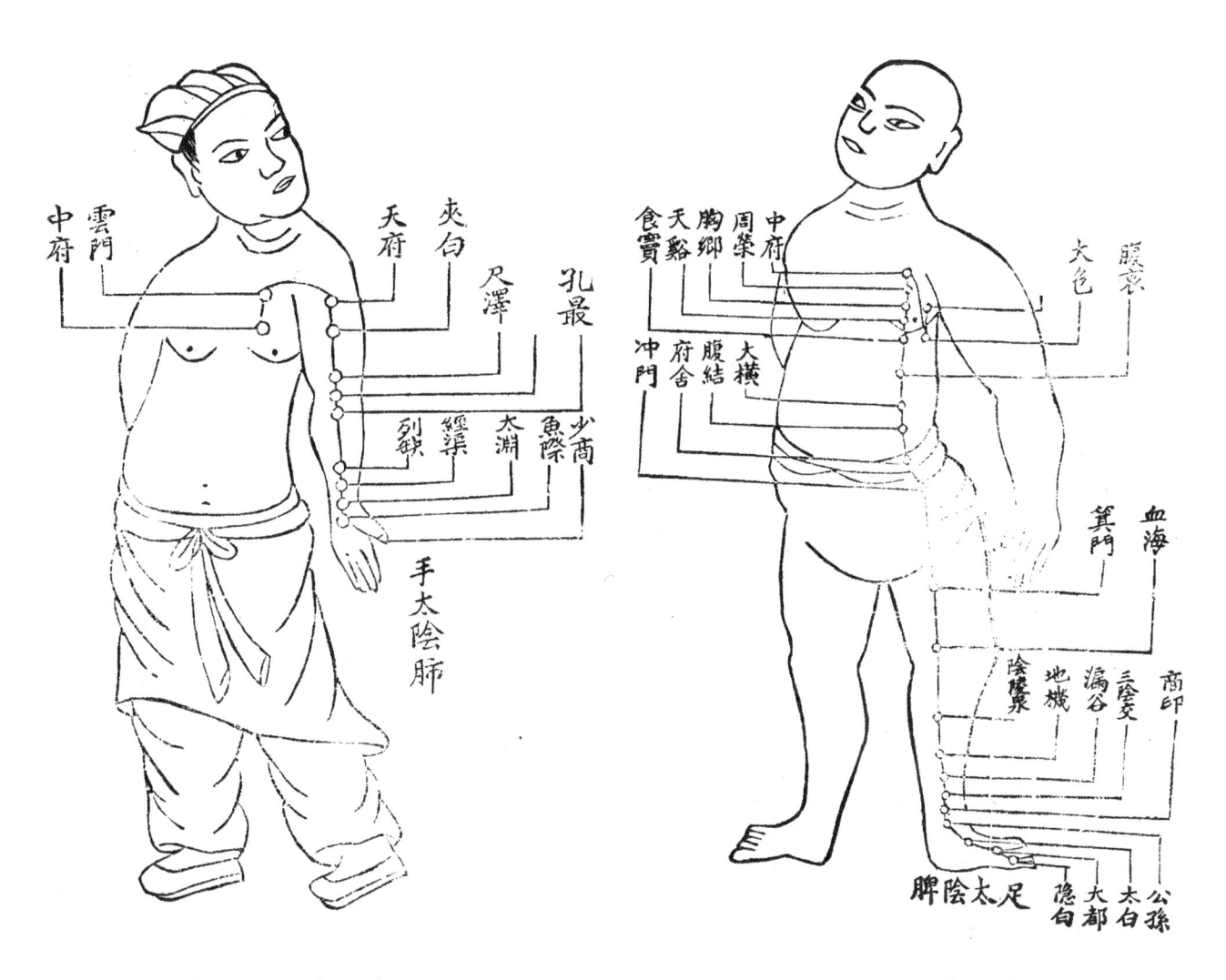

Shou Taiyin [2.4.7]

Zu Taiyin [2.4.8]

THE LITTLE TAIJIQUAN MANUAL FOR BEGINNERS

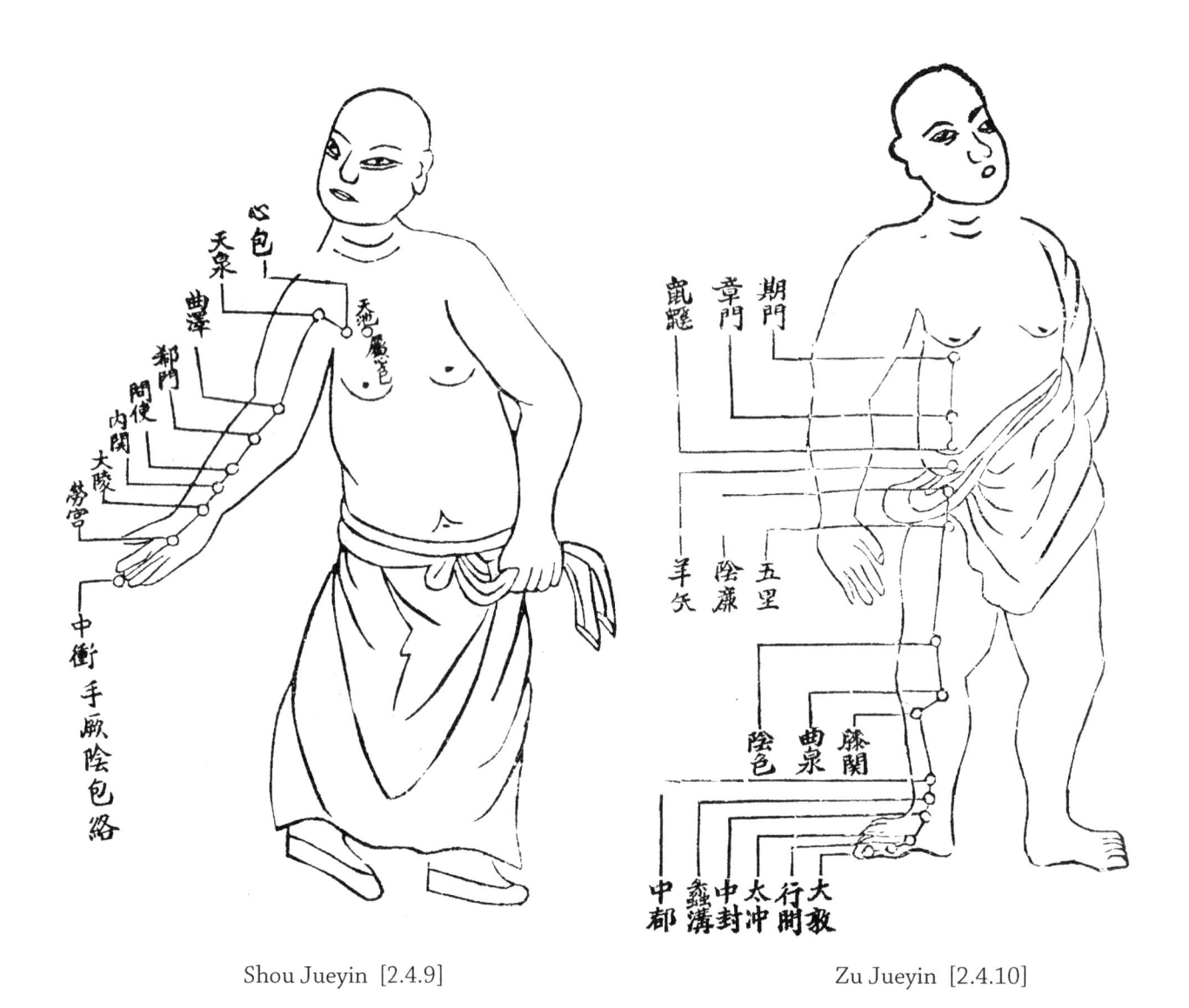

Shou Jueyin [2.4.9]

Zu Jueyin [2.4.10]

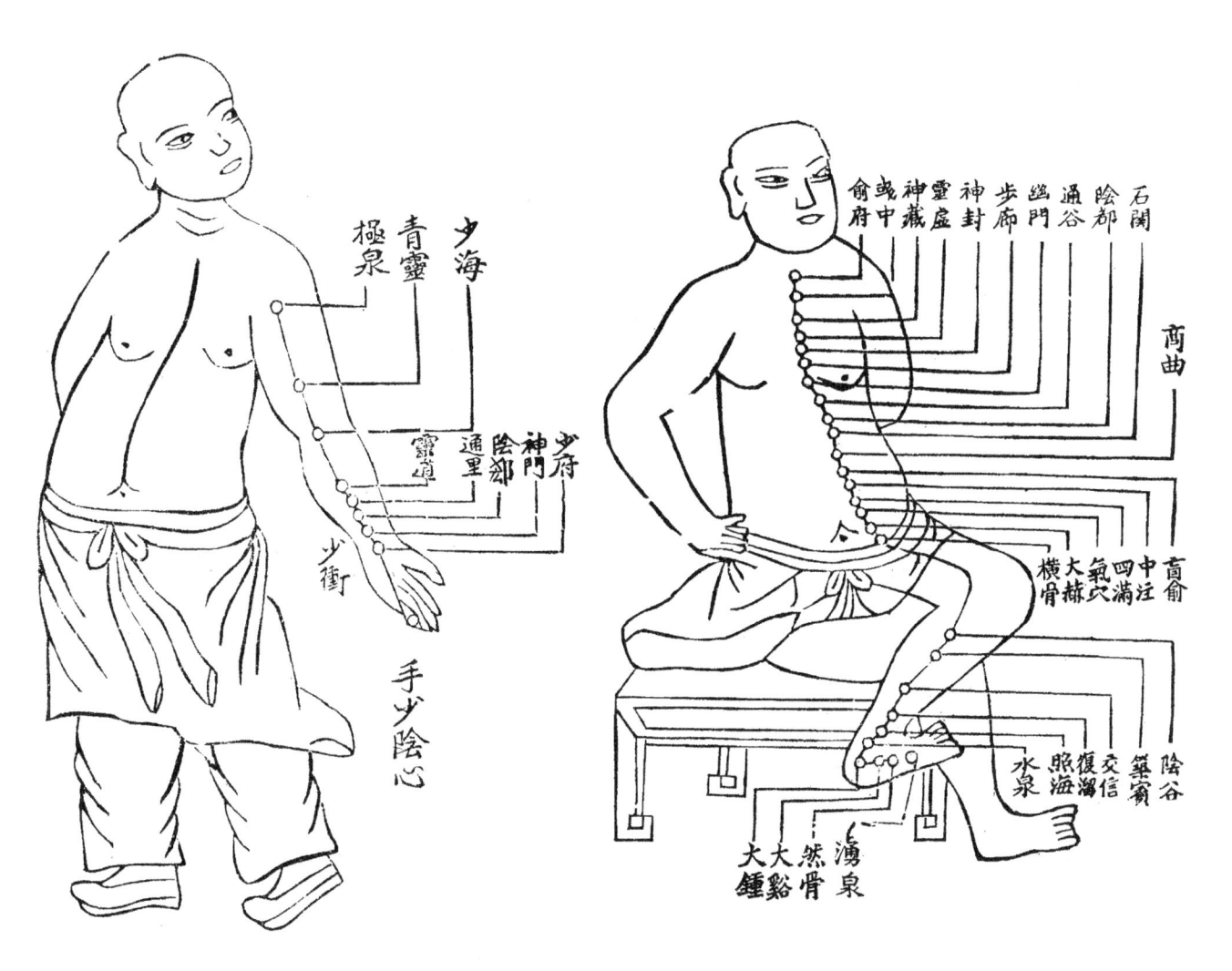

Shou Shaoyin [2.4.11]

Zu Shaoyin [2.4.12]

Renmai [2.4.13]

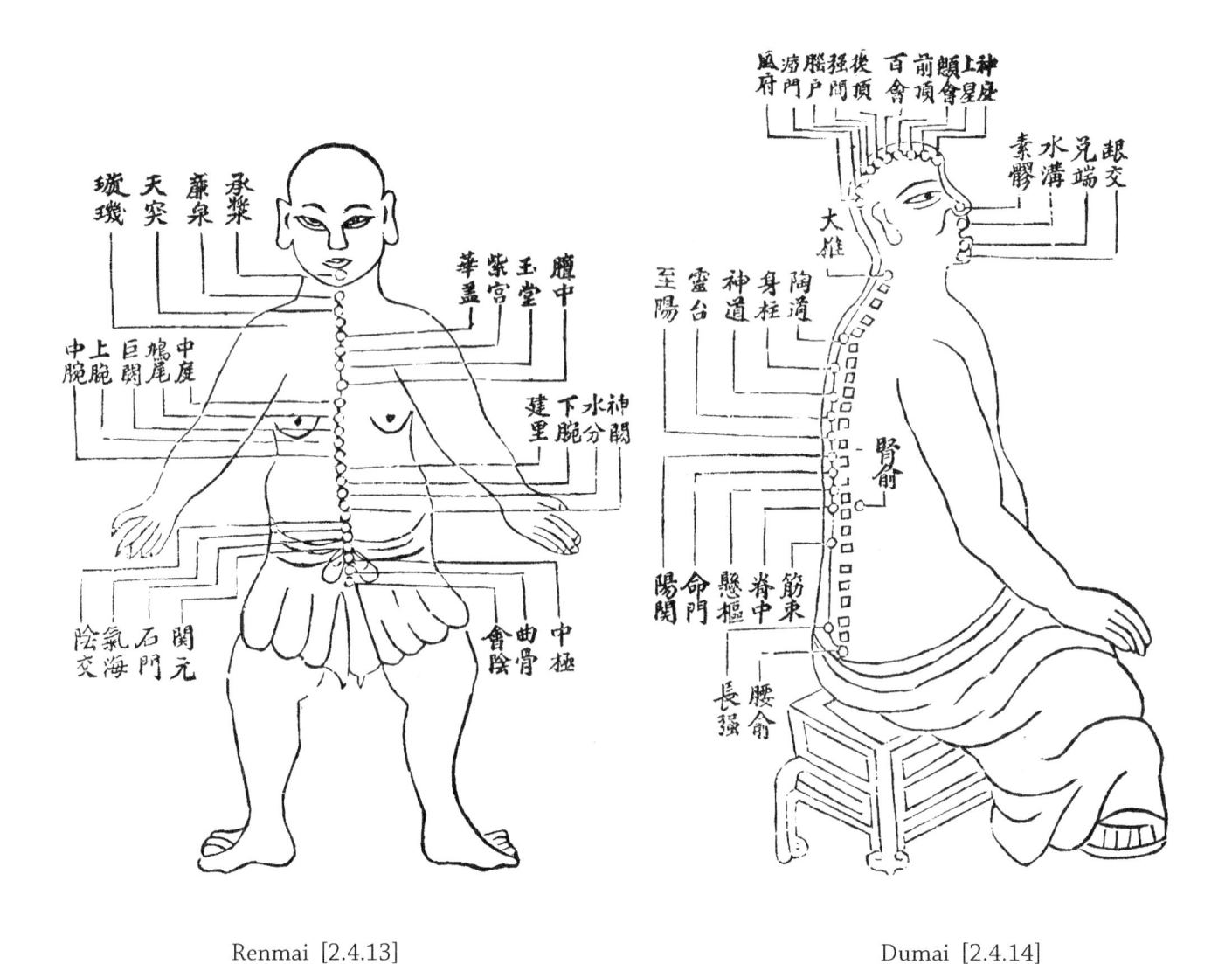

Dumai [2.4.14]

A complete system

Taijiquan is a complete training system. It is self-sufficient, as its content includes but is not limited to: a method for generating mechanical power, application-specific training, traditional weapons training, systematized didactics, a theory of its own, and philosophical foundations. It completely dispenses with any additional training, Chinese or otherwise.

A METHOD FOR GENERATING POWER
Taijiquan is structured around a specific way of generating power, which involves recruiting the deep musculature, making it strong, and optimizing the power transfer throughout the entire body. Muscles and tendons that are barely affected by ordinary exercises will be exercised and strengthened and you will be trained to use them naturally when carrying movements out. There is a simple, objective and effective method to teach the body this skill. It consists in relaxing as much as possible while at the same time keeping the correct posture, which is finely adjusted by the teacher. This training's effect is changing the way your body supports itself and moves. Precisely for this reason, adding extraneous exercises is not only unnecessary, it can be counterproductive for your learning, as you would perform those exercises using your usual way of applying power, the very way you are trying abandon in favor of a new way. Practicing other martial arts systems is even more counterproductive for your Taijiquan learning, as the way you use your body to generate power in those systems would be different. Even other internal arts employ their own particular methods, which are different from Taijiquan's own way.

APPLICATIONS TRAINING
It is very common that the student be anxious to learn applications for the movements in the form, and be frustrated with the delay in getting to this point in practice. Seeing such applications being taught to no avail is likewise all too usual. The movements' practical applications are not at all surprising for anyone familiar martial arts. There are dozens of books available teaching different locks and strikes, all of them useless if the student does not know how to generate power. Incorporating foreign martial training material into Taijiquan is also useless, as Taijiquan is only effective insofar as correct posture and the relative position of the body allow the generation of power, as it is power that makes an application effective.

AEROBIC TRAINING

Aerobic training (cardiovascular conditioning) is a frequent concern of the inexperienced learner, as the traditional way seems slow and the aerobic heartbeat range frequency is not reached. Concern is not warranted because of two facts: first, the slow form of Taijiquan is considered a moderate-intensity cardiovascular exercise, which, in addition to being healthy, covers the needs of most people[1]. Secondly, the slow form normally seen in squares and parks is not the only one. Taijiquan includes a second form called Paochui, which is practiced at high speed and comprises an abundance of jumps and explosive movements. It just happens the vast majority of students does not reach the necessary skill needed to start learning it.

STRETCHING

Regular stretching exercises have limited application for Taijiquan beginners. In order to stretch the muscles the correct way, keeping correct posture and good joint alignment is imperative. Simply trying to stretch yourself as much as possible doesn't come close to that. Additionally, Taijiquan postures that seem to require a lot of stretching are actually difficult to perform not only because of stiffness, but mostly because the student lacks the strength required to keep the correct alignments. Time will be better spent if used to practice forms, and flexibility will increase naturally and gradually. Taijiquan incorporates postures promoting flexibility by design.

QIGONG EXERCISES

Exercises going by the name of Qigong exist in great variety in the repertoire of Chinese body techniques. There are Qigong exercises for almost every imaginable purpose, from activating glands in one's body to stimulating the mental process of meditation, to exercises aimed at developing skills such as breaking stones or making various body parts strike resistant. These exercises can be done without and are foreign to Taijiquan's system, and most of them can be detrimental to practice, a few of them even detrimental to one's health. Taijiquan made ancient combat forms, from which it inherited much, "softer" externally but stronger internally. Taijiquan made power generating methods that existed before its creation "softer" and indirect, and the fruition of practice resulted slower, but much more intense. Taijiquan did the same to martial Qigong exercises. Direct and "hard" Qigong methods were incorporated and made "softer" and indirect, but with a stronger result, even if it took longer. When practicing Taijiquan, one naturally practices proper Qigong. Practicing any Qigong exercise outside the system, even if compatible, actually means a throwback to methods that Taijiquan has improved and made unnecessary or outdated.

CONCENTRATION AND MEDITATION

Likewise, practicing any kind of meditation or concentration exercise as an accessory to Taijiquan practice is not necessary. The training in mental concentration and in enhancing the natural link of mind and body – one of the many reasons Taijiquan is sought after today – is naturally integrated into the system. In a very simple way in fact: a great deal of mental presence is needed to change the way the body moves and generates power, and inner silence and concentration are all the more necessary the more one improves in practice. Concentration ability gradually increases as the body's ability increases. Correct understanding and application of practice method naturally creates concentration and union of mind and body, just as power is naturally generated from the body's correct posture.

This is not to say, however, that practice of sitting meditation is incompatible with Taijiquan - on the contrary. Those already practicing sitting meditation will enjoy many advantages when they start practicing Taijiquan.

SIMPLIFICATIONS AND MODERN DIDACTICS

There is a minimum level below which it is not possible to simplify the system. A few generations ago, the most basic training available was repeating Laojia's first enchainment (Yilu) to exhaustion. Texts by various Masters and oral tradition speak of repeating the form a minimum of ten thousand times to get acquainted with it. If the student were to train the form ten times a day, which means around 4 hours of daily training, and if they practiced every day, it would take them 3 years to have a basic understanding of it. This is clearly too stringent a requirement for most people nowadays. Grandmaster Chen Xiaowang created modernized didactics aiming at meeting current demand for less spartan discipline. However, it is not possible to simplify practice to the point of doing only the the arms' movements, for example, as this would counter a fundamental principle of Taijiquan.

HOW TO PRACTICE TAIJIQUAN

If you want to learn Taijiquan, practice Taijiquan. As obvious as this statement may seem, it is necessary, as it doesn't seem like slow and gentle training like Silk Reeling or Laojia Yilu will make you strong and fast. But if you are under proper guidance, it will become clear very early on that training feels soft but is physically heavy, and any exercise outside the system is a waste of time that should be invested in training in your ultimate goal: Taijiquan itself.

MORE ON ACCESSORY EXERCISES

It is important to understand the above instructions are an expression of a traditional point of view. It is however necessary to take into account who is enunciating them. When a Chen family Master says that you don't need to stretch, as Taijiquan already stretches your body, we must remember they were raised to be a Taijiquan Master. From childhood through adolescence they probably practiced a few hours every day, keeping their body's natural flexibility. They are right in their point of view but their frame of reference is very different from someone who worked for 20 years in an office, and at age 40 decided to start learning. It may be desirable to practice some stretching and mobility exercises. When I was in China for the first time, in 1992, people were used to waiting for their buses in a squatting position - even in Beijing. They would squat for 15 or 20 minutes, with the soles of their feet on the floor, chatting along like it meant no effort. Squatting down fully was resting for them. Compare that to the mobility most people have in their hip joints. Stretching can also be good strategy for gaining mental access to body areas that have long been neglected. When you consciously stretch a body part with which you don't usually work, you cause a feeling there. The feeling of stretching these areas is equivalent to what is called "arrival of Qi" in Chinese Medicine, that is: the first mental access and the increase of blood supply and vitality. On the other hand, some caution is advised. For example, for an elderly person, depending on how sedentary their lifestyle is and how much balance they have, it may be unwise to do certain stretching exercises, both because of the risk of falls and because of the difficulty in keeping a good posture. In cases like these, it may be better to wait up to a few years until stretching is advantageous.

The issue of using weights to increase power is also a delicate one. It will take many years, perhaps more than a decade, before someone starting in Taijiquan will have something to gain from lifting weights, as one first needs to have very a good posture, and be very stable. There are several ways for increasing strength and explosiveness in Taijiquan, including training with traditional heavy weapons, before using weights would be recommended. As mentioned before, if someone uses weights before modifying their body mechanics, they are only reinforcing old mechanics, which they should abandon. That being said, it is possible that, with good guidance, specifically aimed at learning Taijiquan rather than meeting high load goals, and mainly using light loads, some specific weightlifting exercises can be used as a means of encouraging arrival of Qi and its perfusion.

Taijiquan Practice

Values

Taijiquan is an art, and the traditional way of teaching is based on a master-disciple relationship. This does not mean that everyone teaching Taijiquan needs to be a Master, nor that you must become a disciple to practice, even if your teacher is an actual Master (which is very, very rare). We are talking about the relationship's mode, not about technical qualifications or formal positions. A master-disciple relationship means more nuances are present than in a mass education system. As mass education is the system we got used to in school or extra-curricular courses, some points about how teacher and student relate in Taijiquan should be mentioned. There are many legends, sometimes portrayed in films, about how this relationship begins and unfolds. The subject is usually exaggerated or mystified, as is common in movies. It is worth pointing out, however, that when someone is accepted as a student, it is their attitude, character, and willingness to learn that is generally assessed - not their technical proficiency. After all, a student is there for learning, not for demonstrating they already know something.

Over the past 20 years, I have been fortunate enough to live with my Shifu, Chen Yingjun, on several occasions, sometimes for an extended period of time, outside formal class environment. His wife sometimes tells him, "you are from a thousand years ago". It is a compliment that applies not only to his devotion to the art he inherited from his ancestors, but also to his values and personality. On countless occasions, I have seen him put his moral principles above everything else, and my own well-being above his own and above personal gain. It took me a while to realize this, probably because it is so rare these days. He is such a generous person - and not only in the way he teaches Taijiquan - that every time he noticed I was about to take some course of action or say something that would be a clumsy mistake in Chinese culture, he cared to warn me about it before I did. He overlooked my mistakes countless times. Living with him enriched me so much as a person.

LOYALTY
Loyalty is a rare quality these days. When you find a good teacher, be loyal to them. Loyalty doesn't need to be eternal or unconditional: the teacher also has obligations to their students, including being loyal in the same way. It is important that if a departure ever occurs it be clean,

and clear as to when it happens, so that a teacher-student relationship that was once fruitful may become a long term friendship. Loyalty between teachers and students, and among peers, allows a cohesive community to be built, one which will eventually become a school.

PROPRIETY

Taoism, while an important influence in the creation of Taijiquan, was not the only one. The importance of Confucianism in shaping Chinese society and its culture cannot be exaggerated. One of the central concepts of Confucianism is the Rectifying of Names, that is, that everyone has their role in society. A role need not be fixed, but if harmony is to be preserved, each individual needs to know their place and how to conduct themselves accordingly. This means the teacher should behave as teacher, the student as student, the host as host, and the guest as guest. Since we are dealing in a culture very different from the Western one, we should be constantly aware of the expectations in that culture of those in our roles. We must adjust as necessary, as opposed to expecting the culture we are immersing ourselves into adjusts to us. The recent appearance of social media has caused a sudden surge in the number of "masters". This is in stark contrast with what Chinese culture considers proper behaviour. I have lost count of the times I have witnessed my Shifu, Chen Yingjun, an heir of then Chen clan, stop people from calling him Master - interrupting them on the spot, and saying: "my father is the Master". It is a very traditionalist reaction, which I respect and abide by. The concept of Master might, on the other hand, be slightly more flexible. I wouldn't hesitate in stating Chen Yingjun is a Taijiquan Master, as are several of his cousins in the twentieth generation in his family. The number of "masters" we can find nowadays in social media, however, is surely a bit inflated.

DEDICATION

Chen Yingjun once told me:

Dedication sums it up.

There are few people able to devote themselves so completely to a goal as he is, in any field. The required sacrifices are too many, and too big. On the other hand, most people's availability, mainly in taking care of themselves , has been somewhat reduced these days. A little more dedication to one's own well-being and health wouldn't hurt. If there is a certainty in Taijiquan it is there are no shortcuts, the benefits each one receives are exactly proportional to their dedication.

HONESTY

In any honest relationship, sincerity in purpose is essential. A teacher's recommendations to the student should be guided exclusively by the goal of teaching the student to the best of their ability at all times. There should be no hidden agendas. The teacher's influence over the student should never be used for purposes other than the student's improvement.

There should be no secrets about the technique under any circumstances. Once someone is accepted as a student - which presently simply means they have been allowed to attend classes - the practice system must be taught to that person in its entirety. If a teacher does not wish to teach a student, they should not allow their attendance and never collect their tuition. Any deviation from this behaviour is unacceptable. Even implying they are keeping secrets from a student is very offensive for a teacher worthy of the title, as it is the moral equivalent of swindling. If it were not so, trusting the teacher would not be possible for the student, as much as it is necessary for learning. Any Taijiquan student has no idea what they are doing in the first years. Choosing a teacher is almost a leap of faith, as judging a professional's proficiency is impossible for a beginner. That faith must never be betrayed. The teacher can decide which content to teach and when, but the decision must always be taken in the student's best interests.

A Chen family Master, when teaching - even in a seminar, even if not "behind closed doors" - always does their very best, and strives to impart as much as possible of their knowledge to the students, as time and environment allow.

INTEGRITY

The student should constantly remember that what might be not more than a hobby for them, is the teacher's philosophy and way of life.

Be mindful that the knowledge the teacher is transmitting is priceless. Taijiquan is a shining treasure, which took millennia to be discovered and centuries being refined. There is no assessing its value. When you pay tuition, you should keep in mind you are not buying the knowledge, you are only compensating the teacher's time, simply because society works this way. Even more so because it's impossible to buy knowledge: no teacher can teach Taijiquan, no matter how good they and the student are. All a teacher can do is teach you how to practice, and you will cultivate your Gongfu through practice. That is how your Gongfu is yours. Through practice you will build knowledge, and Taijiquan will become your art. All the while, you stay grateful to the teacher who showed you the path and guided you along it.

In short: wisdom is knowing the right path, and integrity is walking it.

HOW TO FIND A GOOD TEACHER

There are many recommendations on the subject, such as: the teacher must belong to a lineage, they must have such and such certifications, they must have a specific technical level, and even they must be trained in this or that subject. These requirements are useless as guarantee that someone is a good teacher. Being connected to a traditional lineage, or reaching a minimum technical level, is simply the bare minimum. How could anyone teach something they don't know? How could they have learned a deep art like Taijiquan, if not in a traditional lineage? There are no self-taught people in this art, for Taijiquan is the result of centuries of evolution. There is no way to start from scratch and reach any acceptable skill level without highly specialized instruction. Unlike a few years ago, nowadays world renowned Taijiquan Masters travel around the globe imparting seminars regularly. Anyone can attend a seminar, and check whether what their teacher tells them is in agreement with what the Masters teach. The technical side is therefore not too difficult to be gauged. The main requirement for being a good teacher is not skill, however. Skill can be learned, and as said, it is the minimum requirement.

The main attribute of a good teacher is character. Unlike skill, character cannot be learned. A good teacher should put the well being of their students first. Their guidance should always aim at what is best for the student, not what is best for themselves. It is not an accident that the term Shifu in Chinese can be translated as father-teacher. Parents and guardians will easily understand the concept, for good parents and guardians put their children first. A teacher's feelings toward their students need not be paternalistic or sentimental, on the contrary - just like a good parent, they should want their students to be free and independent, to learn as well as possible, in order to become strong and healthy, and they should put their learning before self interest. In practical terms, a good teacher will motivate their students to attend seminars with the Masters in the lineage, so they can see a higher level than their own teacher has. A good teacher serves their students by offering them access to the best knowledge sources. A good teacher guides the student along the path of best learning, and teaches them neither more, nor less, if they go astray. A good teacher does not create mysteries nor invents secrets.

WHAT IS GONGFU (OR KUNGFU)

Not long ago, I took my kids for a ride on a Sunday, and we ended up stopping at an old skateboarding bowl, which was empty. They were inside it running and playing, when a freestyle bike rider arrived. The bowl was a bit dirty: piles of leaves and seeds, a clogged drain and a huge puddle of stagnant water. The cyclist leaned his bike against a fence, got a broom and a dustpan from a nearby kiosk, a large empty plastic bag, a 2 liter PET bottle, and some small empty plastic bottles. It took him an hour and a half to clean the bowl, collecting all leaves in the bag, drying up the puddle by removing the water with the large and the small bottles. He then got on his bike and put on a show that made passersby stop and watch. This was an actual Gongfu lesson.

Gongfu literally means great skill gained through great effort. One can find Gongfu in any art or job, and the term is often used with the meaning of skill. It is really more than just skill: it is the cultivation of love for your art, dedication to it and the development of related values.

Technique, Technology and Principles

When one starts learning, it is natural to devote oneself to memorizing the choreography, the outward appearance of the movements. One must first know how to repeat an exercise - be it a form, be it a Silk Reeling exercise - and then perfect it. Later on comes reaping the benefits. This is true for any physical practice.

Most people tend to ask what are the applications for Taijiquan movements. This is due to an expected lack of understanding. Before some experience is gained, it is commonplace to believe learning Taijiquan is learning a collection of self defence techniques, or else that it is learning a movement technique. It is not so.

Chen Wangting, when creating Taijiquan in the 17th century, didn't simply come up with a collection of the most effective free-hand combat techniques in his time, nor did he merely prescribe a training regimen for making the body move skillfully for a particular purpose, as would be the case, say, of an athlete training for high jumps. Taijiquan's founder created a new movement technology, which amounted to a leap beyond everything that was done before. Chen Wangting abandoned the paradigm of simple physical conditioning, and learning techniques, to go on to merge martial arts with the Chinese knowledge about bodily Qi circulation. This was an important change in the way of seeing the body and its movement, and a revolution in the way of training it, overcoming the view of straining one's body until it can no longer bear it, of obtaining strength directly through brute force, and exhausting it in the process, and replacing it by: following the laws of nature expressed in the body, obtaining natural strength by following the alternation and mutual generation of Yin and Yang, and nourishing the body with energy and vitality in the process. Understanding this is crucial for learning.

PRINCIPLES

Taijiquan's principles can be summarized in three statements. The first one regards the organizing principle of the Cosmos, reflected in human beings and their movement. The second one regards the body's posture, that is, the constraining conditions that define the structure of the physical body. The third one regards movement, that is, how to keep this structure and respect the organizing principle during movement.

1. Naturalness

Taijiquan is Dao reflected on the body's movement. It fully obeys the natural laws of interaction between Yin and Yang, which were enunciated in the previous chapter. No anti-physiological movements are performed during practice, and conformity with each practitioner's body comes before any geometrical norm.

2. Waisanhe

Shoulders and hips connect, elbows and knees connect, hands and feet connect. This is how the human body is connected by the natural circulation of vitality. Even if you had never heard about this, and went to an Acupuncture session to treat a musculoskeletal problem, a good Acupuncturist would select the needling points based on this principle. In Taijiquan, one's body is trained in following this natural organizing principle, and in strengthening and optimizing one's power and movement by building on it. In fact, the complete statement of this principle is called Six Harmonies, because there are, besides the Three External Harmonies, the Three Internal Harmonies (Neisanhe). However, the attainment of the latter depends on the attainment of the former, and describing Neisanhe is beyond the scope of this book.

3. The Centre Leads and the Hands Follow

This is the traditional way of stating it. What it means is the body's centre moves, and the whole body follows. Hands are mentioned specifically because they are at the extremity, indicating that the whole body, all the way to the extremities, follows the centre. "Body's centre" can have several meanings. We should initially think of the body's centre as the region comprising from the top of one's thighs to about navel height - the whole contents of this area, including hips, hip joints, lower abdomen, and the lumbar region, everything. Then, as skill increases, this area can be reduced in size, until the student builds and becomes aware of the Dantian. This is a word from Daoist alchemy, which literally means "the concoction's location", or the place where the elixir is made. The Dantian is located four fingers below your navel, inside the body, not on the skin. There is no anatomical structure that corresponds to the Dantian, but there is an Acupuncture point on the skin, called Qihai. I described the location of the centre of the Dantian, but the Dantian itself is a slightly larger region. However, contrary to what drawings might lead one to believe, the Dantian is not a sphere. It is not something solid, and its movement is not limited to what a sphere would be able to accomplish - the Dantian is, on the other hand, a concentration of your body's vital energy. Concentration of Qi should, and can, only be performed in this region. In very advanced skill levels the student moves the energy in the Dantian, and the body follows it with its own movement.

Didactics

I follow Grandmaster Chen Xiaowang's teaching method as passed down to me by his son, Master Chen Yingjun.

Chen Fake was the first in the Chen clan leaving his family's village to teach Taijiquan. He moved to Beijing, and made his ancestors' art known. His sons were the first travelling to various cities in China for the same purpose, and about 40 years ago Grandmaster Chen Xiaowang started travelling outside China. Taijiquan was taught almost only within the Chen family until Chen Fake. Some students who were not from the family were also trained - always within a quasi-familiar relationship, where the student lived with, or met the teacher daily. The most famous example is Yang Luchan, originator of the Yang style, who lived and worked at Chen Dehu's estate, where Chen Changxing, the 14th generation patriarch, taught his family. Yang Luchan trained for many years, while living in Chen Dehu's house, which is now a museum that can be visited. In such a teaching mode, not many technical explanations are necessary, because a high level Master is constantly accessible. Any questions can be answered just by looking at one's own father or uncle, and by placing the hands on one's father's body and feeling how he moves. Learning is intuitive, for the most part. Chen Fake, in Beijing, taught several students who were not relatives, but he was permanently available: his students were intensively dedicated to learning, and he was always present. In the next generation, although Chen Fake's sons traveled throughout China, travelling was not as intense as today. The Master still spent months or years uninterrupted in one place, teaching, and his availability and that of his students remained large. Chen Xiaowang was the first Chen patriarch to face the challenge of teaching students whom he met only a few days a year. Moreover, most of his students were people who could devote only a few hours a week to practice. This pushed him into creating special didactics, and developing verbal explanations for the principles in Taijiquan. The didactics were refined during three decades of international seminars: the sentences that make up a lesson have been tested and modified in order produce the desired effect on the students. This didactic has been stable for several years now.

DIDACTICS, PRINCIPLES, AND METHOD

It is essential for the success of the learning endeavour that the student be able to distinguish the results they want to achieve from the means they will use to do so. Confusion of method and results causes the student not to follow the prescribed method, and to try to obtain results directly - which is impossible.

Didactics

We call didactics the way teaching is structured. A Taijiquan class is usually divided in three parts, and a fourth part may be added according to each student's interest. The structure is as follows:

- A static meditation exercise, called Zhanzhuang, in which a neutral posture, which degree of physical demand is comparatively moderate, is kept long enough to imprint a memory of this posture on body and brain.
- An exercise with simple, repeating movements, called Chansigong or Silk Reeling, which summarizes the basic movement mechanics one aims to learn. This exercise can be explained in a clear way, with distinct steps, each with unique characteristics.
- A more complex exercise with many variations in movement, all based on the same mechanics. This exercise comprises a long choreography, and is what we call Form, or movement enchainment.
- Finally, an exercise called Tuishou, where two students participate, interacting in varying degrees between competitive and cooperative, in which both are forced to, while moving according to the same mechanics, deal with the other person, that uncontrollable variable.

Practice's progress follows the above outline:

- At first, the single hand Silk Reeling exercise seemed confusing enough. Now, several Silk Reeling exercises become part of the student's repertoire, and are used in developing different expressions of the same principle. One's centre's movement, formerly cultivated on a single plane, is now practiced on a plane orthogonal to the first one, and also three-dimensionally. The transitions between the four steps in the Silk Reeling exercises start to blur and become diffuse, and movement becomes fluid and continuous.
- The Form's choreography is no longer a challenge. A 19 postures form used to seem long, now a 75 postures form seems short. One starts identifying the mechanics trained in the repeating exercises within the forms. One learns their first traditional weapon form, and soon the presence of an object is no longer a novelty, and one can see the same body mechanics being applied in increasingly diverse situations.
- The partner exercise is made more difficult: two hands are used, steps are introduced. Then, the cooperative exercise starts alternating with a competitive version, where students have an opportunity to test their balance.

Principles
Principles are master rules guiding practice, or to put it more tangibly, they are the guidelines we want to be able to perfectly follow after many years of practice. We must think about them regularly, and they define what we do. Taijiquan's fundamental principles were described in the previous section.

Knowing and pursuing them is essential for progress, but they *are not* the method for improving. Enunciating principles for a student as if we were teaching Taijiquan would be like giving car keys to a teenager and saying, "please sit behind the wheel and drive". Principles are the destination you are going to, not the way there.

Method
What we call training method is something the student should concretely do when they practice. So you start practicing today, and the teacher tells you that you must move your body's centre, and your hand must follow the centre. How do you do that? You try and copy the teacher's posture. What should you do then to get your hand to follow your centre? There is a simple and concrete method that must be taught to the student so they can improve in their practice. This method regards exactly how they must move their body, and how they must command their body with their brain when trying to move from the centre. There are three resources a teacher uses for conveying the training method: they must explain it verbally to the student, they must demonstrate it so that the student looks and sees what they are talking about, and they must hold the student's hips with their own hands and guide them so they feel what should be done. Without these three components, it is not possible for a student to improve. A student who merely hears the instructions on the method or the enunciation of the principles is doomed to practice for the rest of their life, without improving beyond a very elementary level, for otherwise reading this book would be enough for learning. A student only watching and copying their teacher's movement will also not be able to improve much, otherwise watching and copying a video recording repeatedly would be enough. Touching and guiding the student's body, the third didactic resource, must be seen as essential in transmitting the teachings. Postural adjustments, and regular and repeated adjustment of the movements, when the teacher holds the student's hips and moves them, is the most personalized expression of a teacher's caring for that student's learning.

COMMON QUESTIONS
The most frequently asked question is about practicing alone. How can I practice on my own if I don't

know how to get my body in a good posture? Isn't it better to wait until my posture is correct before trying to practice on my own? Won't practicing in wrong postures be harmful? These questions are born out of misunderstandings about some facts. The first one is the notion of right and wrong. We are indoctrinated from an early age by an educational system that marks our answers in quizzes as right or wrong. You get passing grades or not, graduate or not, and if you graduate, you believe you know something - until you land on the real world. These notions become inculcated deep within us, and they show up when we deal with something new. Unless you have reached a very high level, like that of a Chen family Master, you cannot say your posture is "correct." When you ask a Master if your posture is correct, and they says yes, they mean your posture is fine for now. Continuous, ongoing refinement is what we are talking about. My student's posture is "wrong" from my point of view - but from my Master's point of view, my posture is also "wrong", although a little less so than my student's. Furthermore, since we are talking about body posture and not techniques, you will be adopting your usual posture whether you are practicing Taijiquan or doing the dishes: your body uses its habitual posture spontaneously, all the time. So, let's suppose your posture is "wrong". You can keep using your body like that while doing anything, or you can dedicate some minutes of your day to paying attention to your posture and try to improve it according to the instructions you received in your Taijiquan class. This is why it is always productive to practice, even if "wrong" - as long as you practice moderately. Additionally, you need to create your own internal reference, in order to learn. If you only practice in class, under the teacher's corrections, you won't have anything to compare with the corrections. Practicing alone is part of the learning process, so you can establish an internal reference, get corrections, and compare what you had been doing with the corrections you receive in class. Then you try to change what you had been doing, set another benchmark, get corrections again, compare again, and so on. This is an important cycle. It's possible to learn Taijiquan to a certain extent only by attending classes, without practicing at home, but it's a much slower process.

Practice load is an important factor to consider. It doesn't matter how many years someone has been practicing Taijiquan for, it matters how many hours one has put in. What's the point of practicing for 20 years if someone practiced one hour a week? Not only the amount of total hours is what really matters, but the density of practice as well. If someone practiced a thousand hours in a year, they put in almost three hours a day, but if it took them five years to practice the same thousand hours, they did just over half an hour a day. I wonder which was more productive? That said, the other side of it needs to be looked at. Let's say someone can practice two hours a week: it's better they do it for half an hour on four separate days, than doing those two hours on one single day. Practice is thus better distributed, and their body will receive the skill development stimulus more frequently.

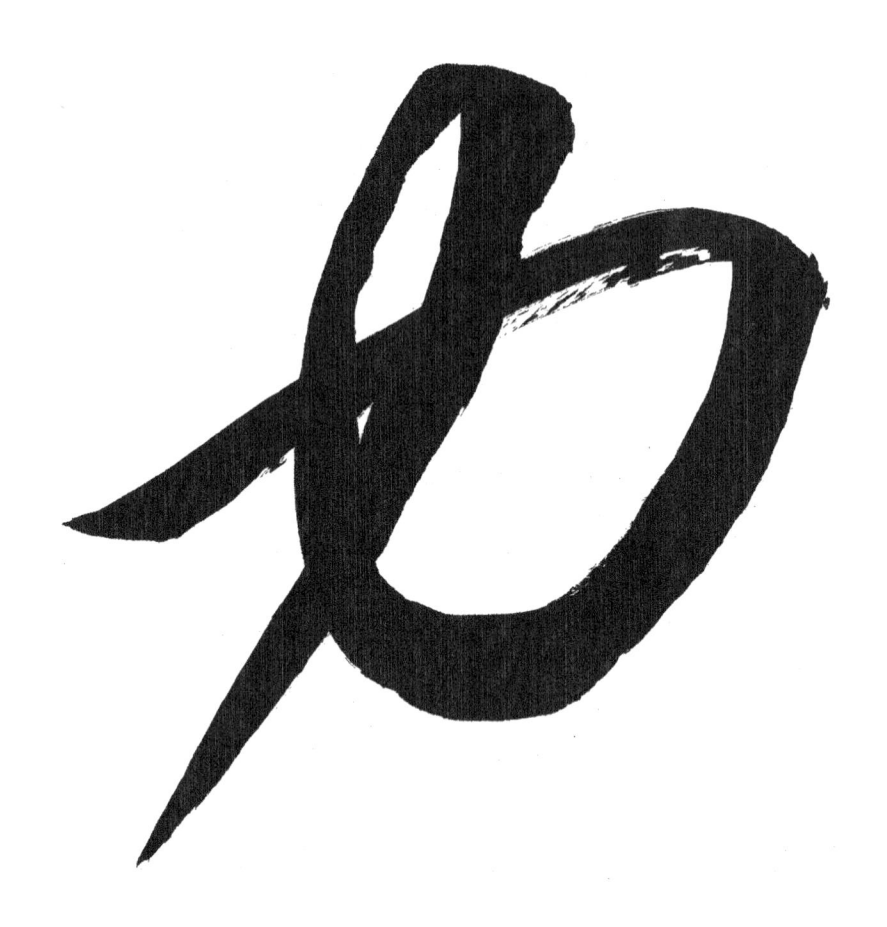

Lì (力): drawing showing the deltoid muscle: strength.

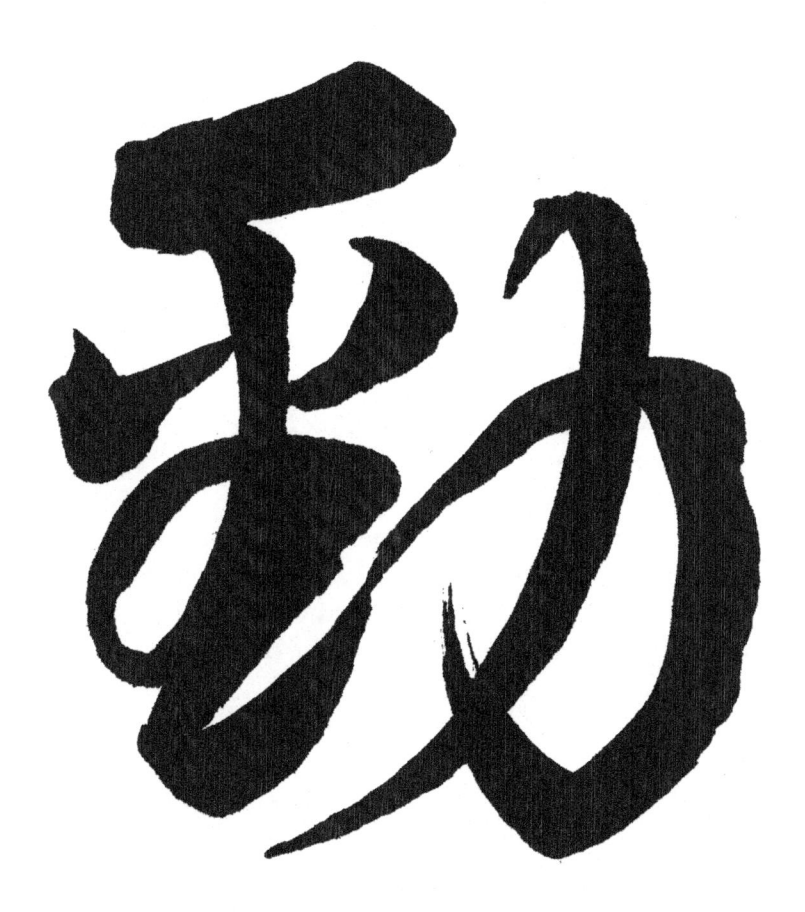

Jìn (劲): on the left side, jīn, the archaic form of "channel", phoneme conveying a sense of flux; on the right, strength: power lì 力 that stretches jīng 经, that follows a line of transmission.

Strength, Qi, Jin, and Qigong

One can use the viewpoint of Yin and Yang to describe countless natural processes. When observing nature in this way, we first see "Yin-Yang pairs," that is, the manifestations of the two opposing principles in any phenomenon. Remembering these principles are complementary, that one does not exist without the other, is important. Asking whether something is Yin or Yang makes no sense, as everything has Yin and Yang within. Is a tree Yin or is it Yang? The crown is Yang in relation to the root, which is more Yin. But the outermost leaves in the crown are more Yang than the innermost leaves, the deeper parts in the roots are more Yin than the uppermost parts.

We can distinguish Yin-Yang pairs in the human body which knowledge is interesting for practicing Taijiquan.

- **Strength and flexibility**

Sometimes we believe we can't reach a given posture because we aren't flexible enough - but after a few months of practicing Taijiquan, without taking time to stretch, we suddenly achieve what we wanted. We acquired enough strength to keep the body in a good posture, and stopped trying to overstretch some of the involved muscles and tendons. Ultimately we acquired more flexibility actually by acquiring strength to keep a better posture. On the other hand, with more flexibility, one is able to keep the correct alignment in a posture at a lower height, thus demanding more power and more muscle recruitment. Flexibility, in this way, allows the generation of even more power.

- **Strength and relaxation**

Telling a student to relax may not be effective in some cases. Someone can only relax if they have enough power. This is the reason why it is easier to relax at a higher posture than at a lower one. It is easy to relax when the load is light. Therefore, the stronger a person is, the more able they are to relax. The more they can relax in a given posture, the more weight they will feel, the more power they will generate.

- **Power and Skill**

If you follow common sense regarding power, and try to get strength for strength's sake by lifting weights, you will soon come across the notion that you need to do sets with few repetitions and heavy loads to increase your strength. Reflecting a little on the mechanics of the exercises would make you wonder what the definition of strength is in such a context. Exercises in these contexts often segment the body, or isolate muscle groups, and the measure of strength is the exercise itself. For example: someone doing exercises for the quadriceps (the muscle group on the anterior aspect of your thighs) on a leg extension table usually measures their strength by the load they can lift in the leg extension exercise, i.e., quadriceps strength would thus be the force delivered at the anterior aspect of the tibia, where the load is applied. This is based on the assumption that if the quadriceps is strong for an exercise isolating it, it will also be strong in other settings - which is not necessarily true. A good counterexample would be proposing that the strength of the quadriceps, developed on the leg extension table, be measured as delivered to the hands in an overhead squat exercise, a squat with the barbell above the head. It becomes obvious then that depending on the context, the word strength can have broader, or less broad, meanings. In the second case above, in addition to the quadriceps being strong, it is necessary that it be so even when the athlete is squatting, and also that its strength be efficiently transmitted to the hands holding the barbell with outstretched arms. It is clear that if we choose this metric, more than just brute strength will be required, and some amount of skill and balance will be needed. What if we choose to measure the force delivered to the hands not vertically, but horizontally? Like pushing a dynamometer on a wall, for example? As we make the measurement requirements more complex, we move closer to the context of actual use of power: the skill of using your power in any direction, at any time, focused and explosively. We then arrive at a mix of strength with the skill of aiming and transmitting that strength, the combination of strength and Qi. We arrive at Qi guiding Li: that's what we call Jin. This Chinese word means something like fluid or refined power, and has special meanings in Taijiquan. It can be accompanied by other terms preceding it, which qualify it and specify its applications. The variations of Jin are usually called 13 Energies or 13 Techniques. The most important one is Pengjin, which refers to the firm and resilient structure, obtained by efficient propagation of the integral force throughout the body.

The last topic is especially interesting. What then is Qigong (or Chi Kung)?

QIGONG OR CHI KUNG

Gong means work, and Qi has several possible translations, one of the most accurate being "vital power". The most popular translation is undoubtedly "energy", which is not a bad translation as long as it's not confused with the concept of energy in Physics. Qigong then literally means "work on vital power". The term Qigong can be applied to any exercise aiming at influencing the circulation of vitality in the human body. Qigong has had many different names in ancient times, such as xingqi (promoting and circulating Qi), fuqi (taking in Qi), tuna (breathing out and breathing in), daoyin (inducing and conducting Qi), shushu (counting the breath), shiqi (living off Qi), jingzuo (sitting still), and wogong (lying down exercise), among others.

In the Zhou dynasty (XI cent. BC to 771 BC) there were inscriptions about Qigong in copper objects, and there is mention of breathing methods in the writings attributed to Laozi (VI cent. BC). In tomb No. 3 of Mawangdui, in Changsha, Hunan province - China, a silk book entitled "On Abandoning Food and Feeding on Qi" and a silk painting with illustrations about daoyin, both from Western Han dynasty (III cent. BC), were found. Classics of Traditional Chinese Medicine such as Neijing Suwen and Zhang Zhongjing's Treatise on Feverish Diseases, both from Han dynasty, expound and suggest Qigong methods to promote health. Since then, renowned doctors like Sun Si-miao, Wang Tao, Li Shizen and Wang An, among others, have mentioned, described and even created Qigong methods.

There are several dozen kinds of different Qigong styles, belonging to different traditions and with different goals. Many of these exercises are beneficial to health and their practice poses no risk, even for frail people; others require a great deal of prior preparation and may even cause harm to the learner if they are not cultivated properly and if detailed instructions that affect one's lifestyle are not followed to the letter.

Qigong and Taijiquan

Taijiquan includes, given enough time and practice, the acquisition of the skill of directing Qi. One can therefore say Taijiquan includes Qigong. Qigong in Taijiquan was learned almost solely within the form up to the 18th generation of the Chen family, by exhaustively repeating forms for years, until the principles of Qi circulation became clear naturally. Chen Xiaowang, taking into account the difficulties of most of his students in implementing such an intensive practice, modernized the spartan didactic, and elaborated basic exercises of Silk Reeling (Chansigong) and Standing Post (Zhanzhuang). We can say that these are the Qigong of Taijiquan, and the principles learned through these exercises should be present during the whole practice.

Taijiquan differs from most Qigong exercises in that no visualization techniques, breath control or mental attention direction (at least for the first many years) should be used to direct Qi. Taijiquan's fundamental principle is naturalness: the way for achieving the skill of circulating Qi is changing the body so it creates conditions for Qi circulation to happen naturally. The body must be trained with Zhanzhuang and Chansigong exercises and with forms, with enough intensity and for enough time so the body's correct posture and movement will allow breath to adjust by itself, and Qi to circulate spontaneously with movement.

Breathing

What I write here applies up to the beginning of the Third Level of Gongfu (read about these levels in the Chapter 4, in the treatise by Grandmaster Chen Xiaowang). There are few people in the world at the Third Level - if you are reading this book, you are almost certainly not one of them. In the Grandmaster's teaching method, forcing one's breath according to any standards is a mistake, for breathing should be natural. As the body is changed, breathing will change spontaneously without need of interference by the student. If one tries to make their breathing forcibly deep, or abdominal, all that ensues is tension. It is necessary to adjust one's posture in the first place, then one is able relax, only then breath automatically and naturally deepens. This is not be controlled by one's will. Taijiquan is not the "martial art of mind control": later on, it is necessary to reach a state of no-mind, of an empty mind, which means there is no mind left that can control anything, there is no "I want" or "I desire", or "I have to".

Qi in Taijiquan

The same goes for Qi circulation: imagining Qi circulation during training is useless, until you have very high skill. Adjusting the body's position and movement with enough precision for the movement to cause spontaneous Qi circulation is the only way to go. Just as it is not possible to push a stronger opponent simply by wishing it very hard, or by concentrating and imagining, it is also not possible to force Qi circulation through concentration or visualizations.

It's very usual that a student starts learning Taijiquan with several misconceptions from previous readings, including "breath power", or "Qi power" and the like. The first expression comes from a mistranslation, mixed with a belief that the Third Level of Gongfu is just around the corner. Sometimes Qi is translated as breath, which is not a bad translation by the way, but it might be the source of confusion regarding breath strength: one confuses vital power with breathing, and one speaks of breath power when one means Qi power. One then believes it is possible to reach the Third Level of Skill after a just few years, when breath synchronization is required during some complex postures in the form. It is not that fast. The second expression, "Qi power", is a myth: there are no shortcuts in learning. An interesting belief once spread in the West: that discovery of a magic force would bring those who practice Taijiquan to suddenly master this art. This belief must have come from some allegory or fanciful story from ancient China. As we have legends and tales in the West, so it is in China. There is no such thing as discovering the "secret" of Qi circulation, and miraculously transforming your body. What actually goes on is training the body through intensive daily practice - so much practice that your body is changed by it - so Qi begins to circulate naturally throughout the body. Still, Qi *guides* the body, or better said, Qi *guides* the body's physical power. It just so happens that when someone practicing Taijiquan reaches sufficient skill to really circulate Qi throughout the body during form practice, making all the circles they should, they are at the boundary of the Second and Third Levels of Gongfu. Someone at this level is already physically very strong, there is already a lot of physical power to be guided by Qi and discharged in a punch or a push. An inattentive observer will not identify this much physical power at first glance, because the appearance of someone at this level is not hypertrophied. On the contrary, it can be misleading.

Chen Zhaopi, one of the exponents of the 18th generation in Chen family, wrote that the first stage in training should be training the body externally by concentrating on the extremities. This stage involved intensive physical practice to "open the joints", and took five years to complete - five years of dedicated daily training under guidance of a highly qualified teacher, and was considered successful when:

- Stomping your foot in Jin Gang Dao Dui has the sound of thunder
- Punching during Yang Shou Hong Quan has the sound of wind
- When jumping in Er Ti Jiao, the kick reaches two and a half meters high [1]

This should be enough to terminate the myth of an ethereal fluid that is capable of causing extraordinary physical effects.

When the average student begins learning Taijiquan, they usually already heard about Qi, and related sensations; on the other hand, they usually carry tension in their body much higher

---

[1] According to David Gaffney's translation

than necessary for their daily tasks. After a few classes and some basic body corrections, they begin to feel and be conscious of the "effects of energy circulation", the most common of which is their hands becoming warm or tingling, or a sensation of heat along the prescribed Qi path in an exercise. The student gets impressed and thinks they can circulate Qi with their will. Shortly after, the effect disappears, the student is disappointed in themselves or the art, and abandons practice. Let's make it clear: if energy did not circulate naturally in your body, you would be dead. The warming effect is nothing more than the increase of peripheric blood circulation due to initial relaxation. The body quickly gets used to the increase, and the sensation disappears.

It will not happen, contrary to what you might think at first, that Qi circulation will get stronger and stronger, and the hands will be hotter and hotter. We are not talking about electricity here. If it were like that, Chen Xiaowang's hands would be continuously on fire. What happens is that you become more and more sensitive, and become capable of feeling and of dealing with smaller and more subtle sensations. An increasingly better circulation of Qi means your movements are more and more precise and refined, and you feel your body with an increasing degree of detail and depth.

TAOIST ALCHEMY
When I first went to Australia and stayed at Chen Xiaowang's house to learn from Chen Yingjun, his son, I had been practicing Microcosmic Orbit on my own, a well-known Taoist exercise, for quite a while. The exercise is performed in a sitting pose, and one imagines Qi going up the spine and down the front of the body (with a few more technical details). I was already used to the exercise and practiced it for about an hour a day. I had already consulted some experts on the subject, and heard there were "secrets that were revealed only to initiates" and "secret keys" to ensure the effectiveness of the exercise. In the evening of receiving Chen Yingjun's first postural corrections to my Zhanzhuang, I practiced Microcosmic Orbit in my bedroom. The result was shocking, I had never felt anything that strong. On the second evening the effect was the same. It was obvious to me that the improvement was caused by the postural corrections, and I abandoned the Microcosmic Orbit to practice only Zhanzhuang.

On another occasion, I asked Chen Yingjun if I should try circulating Qi in the above described way. He replied, "Don't worry about it, it will happen naturally during the form, when your skill is better". Today, twenty one years later, I am a witness to that.

TAIJIQUAN MASTERS, AND TUISHOU

There really are effects that seem inexplicable when you practice push hands with a real Master. Chen Yingjun, for example, has shown me several times he can make me stand on my tiptoes, just by touching my armpit with his forearm. He has shown it very slowly - in slow motion - and even stopped midway. How could this be possible? When he throws someone meters away, his sheer power explains what he does. But how can one explain it, when he barely seems to exert any pressure? A student of mine likes to quote Arthur C. Clarke: "Any sufficiently advanced technology is indistinguishable from magic".

The Japanese Neurologist Yoshio Manaka was a genius in his generation. He became a world-renowned Acupuncturist, and created absolutely original - and amazingly effective - treatment techniques that no one following the classics would imagine. He theorized, in his book *Chasing the Dragon's Tail*, that, besides the two main information systems in human body - the Nervous System and the Endocrine System - we would have a primitive information transmission system, which would have been made obsolete by evolution and relegated to the background. According to Manaka, Acupuncture would act on this primitive system, using it to propagate information throughout the body, helping its self-regulation. Although Manaka's theories have not inspired further research and experiments to prove them, we can think about how they would be reflected in Taijiquan. Let's start with a professional boxer: sometimes we see a beginner boxer having trouble landing a punch because his body movement announces beforehand what he is going to do. We say that a bad boxer telegraphs his punches. A good boxer takes advantage of this phenomenon, throwing punches without telegraphing them, or falsely telegraphing different punches than he is actually going to throw, in order to mislead his opponent. A good Judo fighter can do something similar, while touching the opponent, in this case up close, using the opponent's sense of touch and balance more than their sight. The opponent's reactions, if they are inferior or poorly trained, occur on a subconscious level, and they are totally ensnared. Based on Manaka's Acupuncture theory, and what I described above about Boxing and Judo, I believe that the seemingly magical effects that Taijiquan Masters achieve in Tuishou are somewhere between the two, but at a much higher subtlety level. Taijiquan offers a systematic means of developing these skills beyond what would be possible only intuitively. When a Master manages to uproot an opponent by merely touching him, seemingly not using the physical force necessary for the feat, he's not really using only force - he's manipulating the unconscious information system feeding that person's sense of balance.

This causes something like a blockage, or an information flooding in that system, making it impossible for the person to readjust their position in time to keep balance, and they have a feeling of distress and repulsion, losing the ability to react effectively. Starting from where the martial arts of his time were, Chen Wangting, through his new movement technology, was able to greatly refine how someone's highly trained body influences an opponent's body movement.

I'm adding something new here. I formerly said Qi circulation is a measure of the Taijiquan student's skill in transmitting spiralling power through their body. It is not just force being transmitted, information also is.

This is only logical. The nervous system is at the centre of it all, with information actually being transmitted to and from the brain, but I'll simplify the picture a little. As mechanical force is being transmitted from the centre of the body, through the joints on its way to the fist, information about position and force is also being transmitted. When starting to learn this is done consciously, and is therefore ineffective. With time and repetition, as the student moves their Dantian and begins to spiral muscles and tendons above and below it, they feel the spiral and dynamically regulate the intensity of torsion and the synchronization to it in the next part of the body - hip, torso, shoulder, elbow, up to the hand. If the torsion and extension of limbs is at a greater or lesser speed than ideal, the circulation of energy is less than optimal. This "feeling and regulating" is the transmission of information. Without question, this must come about spontaneously, unconsciously. If the student tries to twist and regulate the body with excessive presence of mind and will, they will achieve nothing but a robotic appearance. This shows how the "relax" instruction is all important. I must stress that the above description is solely a theoretical discussion, not a prescription for practice. This is not the way to practice, for this is not the method of training. This is also why instructions like "use" or "engage such muscles" are insufficient, and almost always inappropriate, for teaching and describing Taijiquan. We need, as I said before, a language with a higher level of abstraction - the language of Qi.

When a Master corrects your posture during a seminar, you are faced with a question: How is it possible that they adjust my position with such precision? How can the physical effort after the adjustments be so intense, and at the same time I feel so comfortable? How were they able to move and activate deep layers of my musculature, touching only my skin? The explanation is above. If the Master masters their own body as I explained, they can influence the student's body to the same extent. The situation is in principle the same against an opponent, but the opponent is trying to go against it, at high speed.

Fengshui

Fengshui is the Chinese knowledge about locating and positioning in relation to the environment. In our case, the applications are quite simple. You can practice almost anywhere. I have already spent a month living in a budget hotel room that had only a one-by-two meters space where I could move, and I practiced every day, two hours a day. It's a far less than ideal condition, and it does interfere with results - but there are still gains. The ideal place for practice is flat and close to nature. A forest or a park is great. It needs to be more or less peaceful: there should not be excessive noise or too many people around, as this hinders relaxation and concentration. The perfect place would have a nearby stream, with that soft running water noise in the background, and your back should be turned its way. In warm countries it is best to practice in the shade. Everyone feels better at place like this, with trees and fresh air. It has been proven that noise causes stress, it is important then to have some measure of silence. People who live in noisy places have more cortisol in their saliva than people who live in quiet places - salivary cortisol is linked to stress. If there are too many people around, one's sense of self-preservation will not turn off. Every animal needs a minimum territorial area for feeling safe, and if this area is breached, aggression results. Human beings, although they are sociable and live under norms of civility, are still subject to self-preservation biological reflexes, and how much you can relax is linked to it. If you are alone - without a teacher who's in charge of caring for the practice area - it may be better for Zhanzhuang to be done at home, in a quiet room, than in a park. It is very hard to relax with your eyes closed in a public place, when you are by yourself.

 It is best to avoid uneven or slanted ground. You are trying to regulate your body's sense of structure and vertical alignment, and any complicating factors will make your job more difficult. Shoes with slanted soles should be avoided. Rectangular places help maintaining a sense of direction. If the site does not have rectangular boundaries, there may be a straight fence, wall, or path that could be used for this purpose. Marks on a room's floor, such as tile seams or running boards, can be used as precise references. I used a string stretched across my living room's floor, until I built a solid enough internal reference. It is often said that mirrors are not very useful. Using a mirror however, specially to one's side, has been very useful to me for quite some time. You can check if your body is vertical, and you can see something about your hips' position and your spine's shape. I had a mirror framed and hung on the side wall of my living room, so to keep track of my posture, during a long phase of my apprenticeship. On the other hand, it is desirable that at a certain point in your progress you abandon the mirror and create a completely internal sense of alignment. This does not have to be done in a day; if you have been using a mirror as an aid, it is better that you abandon it gradually, when you decide to do so. For example, you could reduce the use of the mirror to the point when you look at it only once a month.

A common question students have is about the best time to practice. There is, in theory, a better time to practice, but you don't have to worry about that. The answer is simple: the best time is the time you can make it. With our busy life these days, setting aside half an hour a day to take care of yourself is a feat. On the other hand, someone like Chen Yingjun, practicing professionally, dedicating 6 to 8 hours a day to this, doesn't even think about the question of a better time in the day. He practices all day long, pausing for meals only. When Taijiquan arrived in Brazil, where I was born, most people believed that one had to practice close to sunrise. This was just a circumstance, because pioneer groups practiced in public parks, and it's usually too hot under the Brazilian sun, even at 7am. In Germany, where I trained in winter, outdoor practice was between 10 am and 4 pm, when the sun was warmest.

The clothes you choose are not too important, it is enough that you feel comfortable, and clothes do not hinder your movements. Footwear, on the other hand, should be suitable. Choosing good shoes for practice can be a difficult task, and Taijiquan people usually become shoe nerds. The main requirement is that the sole be flat; running shoes with thicker soles on the heel are not advised, as they change one's balance, and hip and spine positioning. Besides having a completely flat sole, ideally shoes should be light and flexible, and if possible should have a wide toe box, so the toes are not squeezed.

Some ancient texts used to recommend practicing Taijiquan facing south, and gave instructions on posture directions using cardinal points, taking south as the starting position. If you live in Wenxian in winter, when it's -12°C and there's no heating inside, you'll understand on the first day that you'll freeze if you don't practice facing the sun, which is always south because of latitude. If you live in southern Chile, and practice outdoors in winter, you should face north. Unlike in China, in Chile the direction of light - where sunlight comes from - is north. It is better to hide from the scorching sun in a tropical country, on the other hand. If you are just starting to learn, it is a good idea not to practice in places where it is too windy, especially not Zhanzhuang. With strong wind there are usually gusts, and it can be difficult to concentrate and even keep your balance in rapidly varying wind direction. It is unpleasant to train like this, and sometimes unproductive. It is traditionally said that "wind scatters Qi".

When Taijiquan came to the West, practicing with music became a widespread habit. The best music is silence, or the sound of a distant stream, as said before. Relaxing music can be useful to hide background noises disturbing your peace - if you have bothersome neighbours, there's nothing wrong with using light music to drown their noise.

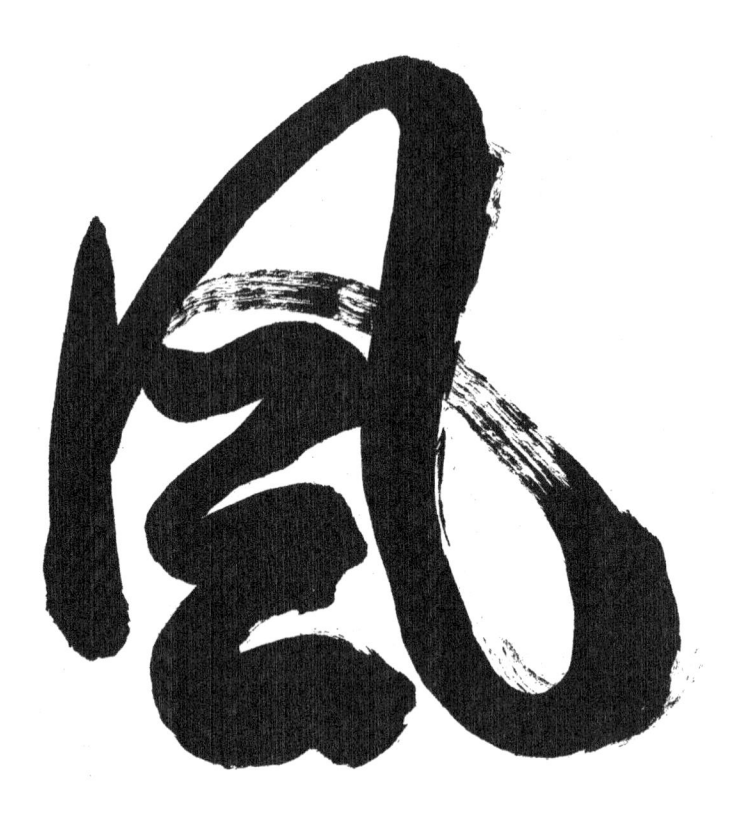

Fēngshuǐ (風水): fēng 風, wind, and shuǐ 水, water: Chinese geomancy, a doctrine aiming to determine the flow of energy in a space, in order to better adapt human presence to its qualities.

水

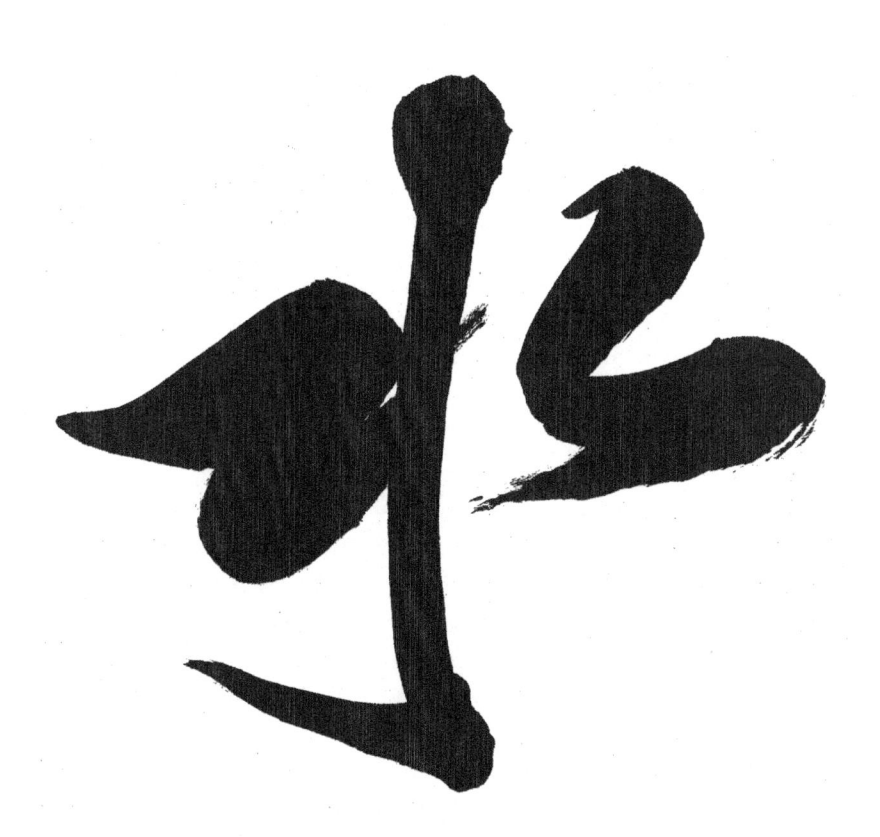

Body positioning

Geometric rules regarding body posture should be avoided because they do not take into account the enormous anatomical variation among people. It is very usual to see new students trying to apply geometric rules they have heard or read somewhere else to their bodies, at all costs. When I write "at all costs" I mean that many people abandon basic logic, perform flagrantly anti-physiological movements, bear joint pain, and keep believing arbitrary rules which origin they don't even know.

Some rules are created to simplify explanations, or almost accidentally, when there is no time for detailed descriptions, as in a class for a very large group during a seminar. A good example is when someone says the feet must be parallel in Zhanzhuang. How could they be parallel, if they are not even regular geometric shapes? Which edges should be parallel, the inner or the outer edges? In fact, none. The feet should be, in most cases, simply in a symmetrical angle in relation to where one is facing. One's toes may be open more or less visibly, depending on that person's hip joints and postural habits.

Some rules are created to try and avoid accidents or injuries. An example is when someone says that the knees should not go beyond the toes during practice. This is true only in a few cases, particularly when the posture is high. However, for low postures, such as The Dragon Lays Down to the Ground, it is an impossible rule to follow - the knee will go beyond the toes, and by how much depends on the size of the femur, and its size in relation to the body.

Still other rules are created by an unfounded assumption, and are grave mistakes. The worst of them is "tucking the tailbone", a concept that didn't exist in Taijiquan until the 50's. In the following decade, some books in Hong Kong adopted, for no apparent reason, the erroneous idea that the hip should be posteriorly tilted, or the tailbone tucked forward. This concept must be forsaken, for it's a gross mistake and causes serious problems.

Whatever the case, standards such as these do not take into account every individual's anatomical variations. If you saw how much variation is possible in shape, size, and angle of the human femur's head and neck, you would be amazed - and that's just one single bone in the body. Geometric standards, however well-intentioned, turn out to be wrong for most people because they are too general.

HEAD

One's head should be upright, that is, it should be vertical. This simply means that it should not hang forward, backward, or sideways. One's neck should remain relaxed, and the neck's physiological curve should not be interfered with. A good reference is looking to the horizon. During the early years in practice there is a tendency of looking down and checking one's posture and foot positioning. This is not a problem per se, but if one is not careful, it can turn into a habit. No one, when looking down, moves only their head: we all tilt the body a little when looking, thus losing vertical alignment. If, however, we look to the horizon, we have a reliable horizontal reference, and consequently a good sense of the vertical direction. There are often questions about the tongue touching the palate. The standard answer is that this connects Dumai and Renmai (which are energy channels in the human body). This answer means very little in practice. Lightly touching the palate with tip of one's tongue is part of the posture, that is, it helps the muscles in the face and neck area to position properly, which influences the rest of the body. But this instruction is very seldom transmitted by Grandmaster Chen Xiaowang in his seminars, which indicates it is an instruction of little importance for the average student. You shouldn't worry too much about it at first, there are far more important postural adjustments to get right before this one has any significant effect.

SHOULDERS AND ARMS

Shoulders should be relaxed, but when we say this to students, they react according to their usual idea of relaxation, not according to the relaxation they are trying to learn - which is to be expected, as they haven't learned it yet. What then? Shoulders should be "in their cradle", that is, not shifted forward or back. If this is done correctly, the student will have a feeling of light arms, which is in accordance with Yin and Yang, because the arms are high up in the body, which belongs to Yang. If you feel your arms are heavy, your shoulders are possibly shifted forward.

The distance of one's hands to the body during Zhanzhuang and during Taijiquan movements is cause of many misunderstandings. Students see photographs of Chen Xiaowang practicing Zhanzhuang, and try to copy the geometric position of his arms and hands, making a large circle at shoulder height. Without any question, the Grandmaster's posture is correct - actually perfect - but it is so for him, not for the vast majority of students. Chen Xiaowang is very strong, way stronger than one can guess by looking at him. Trying to copy his posture by keeping the same stance height or copying how wide his arms are, is a mistake. It is not possible to copy the Grandmaster's postures while still following all technical requirements, without having his strength. The beginner's hands, during Zhanzhuang, will normally be at about the solar plexus height, and can be as low as the navel if needed, so to allow shoulders and arms to relax.

CHEST

It is said the chest should be empty and the abdomen, or more precisely, the Dantian, full. This does not mean the chest should be depressed or compressed downward. If shoulders are slumped forward, the chest will very probably be compressed. If it is so, it may be depressed, or strained upwards in trying to compensate the compression. There is one other complicating factor. Exercise-related magazines, images of superheroes in movies, and the prevailing aesthetic standard all portray men and women with their chests full and pulled upwards, and our tendency is to copy these patterns unconsciously. The problem is intensified by linking a full chest with ideas of pride and virility. All of this should be avoided. It's easy to understand the issue intellectually, but after years doing this unconsciously, we all have a hard time relaxing our chests. Try and analyze pictures of Chen Xiaowang and Chen Yingjun, and notice how they do not fill up their chests, and how the pectoral muscles are not hypertrophied.

SPINE

The spine's shape is one of the concepts causing most confusion for beginners. The confusion is increased by ignoring the spine's anatomy and some basic principles. In a few words: the physiologic curvature of the spine must be respected during Taijiquan practice. It's wrong to try and make the spine, or any part of it, straight.

The spine has four physiological curves: cervical lordosis, thoracic kyphosis, lumbar lordosis, and sacral kyphosis. Every healthy human being has these curves, starting at a certain age - for they become established some time after a child has learned to walk, and has adopted upright posture. The vertebrae themselves are classified by their main characteristics, which are a function of their position in the spine. Vertebrae have two lateral "arms," called transverse processes. At the end of these processes are the articular facets, which articulate with the same facets of the vertebra above and below. Picture this by opening your arms out to the sides: if you were a vertebra, your hands would be the equivalent of the articular facets. The facets's angle varies according to the position of the vertebra in the spine (it's as if you turned your palms up or down a little). This alone would be enough to show that the vertebrae in the spine, which have developed over millions of years through natural selection to reach their current shape, are adapted to the spine's natural shape. In addition, we should mention the vertebrae have a long protuberance on their posterior aspect, called spinous process. This is what you see when you look at a person's back, and notice their spine. The spinous processes come out of each vertebra at a specific angle, which varies with the position of the vertebra in the spine. The vertebrae thus stack and fit together perfectly, and the spine has its natural shape and curvatures. There are two simple deviations of the spine's curvatures: the excess of curvature (hyperlordosis or hyperkyphosis), and the rectification of curvature. If you talk to an Orthopedist or a Physical Therapist, they will tell you that the rectification of a curvature of the spine is a deviation, something that is not healthy and requires treatment. Straightening of the spine's curvatures is as bad as excesses in the curvatures.

Taijiquan respects the natural curves in the spine. Notice that the instruction for a correct posture is "keep the body straight", not "keep the spine straight". Keeping the body straight means not leaning forward or backwards, either with the whole body or with part of it. The fundamental organizing principle in Taijiquan is naturalness. Therefore, the spine's physiology and natural shape must be respected. The hips must be correctly positioned for the spine to be in its natural shape.

HIPS

Until about 1950, according to Jan Silberstorff's research, Taijiquan books in China printed traditional instructions about the hip. From the 60's on, this changed, and books started recommending that one "tuck" the tailbone by posteriorly tilting the hip. This is a very serious mistake. One must not try to forcibly tuck the tailbone or posteriorly tilt the hip when practicing Taijiquan, in no way. It's not known why some books recently started recommending that. Maybe there was some influence from western calisthenics, maybe an isolated opinion became popular. You should know that this absurd idea is in complete disagreement with the traditional instructions transmitted by Chen Family Masters.

Analyzing this error through a logical lens, it is easy to conclude that tucking the tailbone:

- Strains the anterior muscles in the hip-femoral joint, leaving the posterior muscles flaccid and shortened;
- Locks the hip joint, reducing its freedom of movement;
- Prevents the free rotation of the femoral head in the acetabulum, causing the knee to suffer undesirable lateral and torsional loads;
- Reduces the use of the quadriceps, decreasing power in the legs;
- Rectifies the physiological curve in the lumbar spine (which is not healthy);
- Causes excessive wear in the articular cartilage of the hip-femoral joint;

- Stiffens the body, making it a rigid block with reduced mobility;
- Tenses the lower abdominal region, which should be relaxed (although naturally active).

In short, tucking the tailbone is a disaster for a Taijiquan student. From the point of view of energy circulation, tension on the anterior hip and on the lower abdomen hinders the connection between the upper and the lower body. The Dantian area, which should be relaxed to allow deep breathing, will be tense.

How to position the hip correctly
When Chen Xiaowang says "relax the whole body," this is exactly what he means. The whole body should be relaxed, without exception - especially the centre of the body, which commands everything else. It is well known that in a correct posture the gluteal region should not protrude, but the hips should not be pushed forward either - it would be as bad a mistake in the opposite direction. The hip should be relaxed, and loose so as to be able to move. It is not possible to teach this precisely in a book, nor by means of pictures or videos. It is essential to get regular postural adjustments from a good teacher.

KNEES
Leave your knees alone. I could say it in countless ways. A huge number of martial arts students, even Taijiquan students, have had knee problems. Why? Simple enough: wrong instructions, and lack of knowledge. Knees are delicate joints, which work approximately like hinges. It is important to emphasize "approximately". One should not apply lateral loads to the knees, or else risk damaging menisci and ligaments. If you read my short autobiographical account at the beginning, you know I badly injured one knee before meeting the Chen family. It happened because I was following wrong instructions I received while practicing a different style. At the time, I was told the knees should be kept right above the toes on a vertical line, pulling the knees out if need be. This is really bad for joint health. Knees should move naturally. They are capable of transmitting spiral energy and power that flow through the body, but effective transmission should always be obtained by means of relaxing and keeping a good posture, never forcibly twisting or pulling the knees. The hip joints are responsible for most of the twisting in the legs, so, beware: if the hip joints are locked or tense, specially because of the grave mistake of "tucking the tailbone", they will not be free to move, and the knees will suffer undue loads.

It may be useful to have more detailed information regarding the question of knees and feet. The commonly repeated, but incomplete, instruction is that "knees should be in the *direction of* the toes". This is an incomplete instruction because, in order to define a direction, two points are required, and it only mentions the feet - only one point. What would the second point be? Since the knee transmits power, the second point is the area where power is generated: the centre of the body. The centre of the body is however a large volume, not a point, in a context of power generation. The incomplete instruction then becomes an imprecise instruction - the only solution is in person instruction from a knowledgeable teacher who will adjust your posture with their own hands. A Master can enunciate the above instruction in a class, as they will proceed to adjusting the students' posture, supplementing the verbal instruction. Problems often occur when the instruction is heard, but the postural adjustments are not understood. The instruction is then almost always confused with "the knees should be *vertical to the* toes", which is a serious mistake. This last sentence disregards the direction of power through the leg and the spiral in the joints. If you imagine your foot fixed on the ground, and think of turning the body a little towards one side, you will understand all joints in the leg are capable of a little coiling, without creating transversal loads. If the leg is relaxed, and the hip joint is free to move, the knee and ankle will also turn slightly, and coil a little. Additionally, the position of the knees depends on the size of the femur in relation to the rest of the body, and on the angle and size of the femur's neck. Imagine someone squatting: if the femur is longer, the knees will go further over the toes; if the femur is shorter, the knees will go over the toes a little less. The same variations influence any posture, although the influence is not as evident as when squatting.

POSITIONING THE FEET

Feet positioning is also source of misunderstandings for those starting to practice Taijiquan. There are two reasons why: either the student has had previous instruction in another martial art style, or they are worried about the matter. In the second case it's easy to vanquish the questions, just a quick explanation suffices. In the first case, however, it is necessary to explain in detail. Almost all students with previous experience in martial arts tend to follow geometrical rules about the body's posture, and one of the most prevalent is trying to keep the feet parallel during Zhanzhuang. This is a mistake, and is damaging to the joints. One should never try to forcibly position the feet, as all this accomplishes is decreasing freedom of rotation in the hip joints, and - again - causing knees to bear lateral loads. Feet should be positioned naturally.

When teaching someone without previous experience, one usually does not even mention feet position, so as not to interfere with the natural way. For example, when teaching a child, feet are not mentioned. Sometimes, saying the feet should be naturally positioned is not enough. We can then say that feet should *ideally* be symmetrical during Zhanzhuang. This means they should be side by side, not in front or behind each other, and the toes can be slightly open. How much the toes should open out depends on each individual student, but they should normally be open the same angle, not one of them more open than the other. These instructions, however, do not apply to all people, they are idealized. If someone has a hip deviation which is a little larger than commonly found, these instructions no longer apply: therefore, the best instruction is positioning the feet naturally.

Zhanzhuang

Grandmaster Chen Xiaowang included an exercise in his didactics with which we start every class, and which practice is essential for changing the body and learning Taijiquan. Its Chinese name is Zhanzhuang. Good translations would be: pillar posture, stake or pole posture, or standing like a pole, or standing meditation. The Chinese characters for Zhanzhuang convey the idea of stability, and this is the main concept.

There is a prescribed method for entering this posture, with physical and mental procedures, developed by Chen Xiaowang to induce the beginner in obtaining the benefits of its practice. Verbal instructions are given before the teacher begins the postural adjustments:

1. Calm down. Keep your head upright, keep your body straight (top of your head, ears, shoulders, hips, and ankles, in the same vertical plane).

Keeping the head upright simply means keeping it vertical. There is a traditional instruction saying that "the top of the head should be light as if suspended by a thread", but this does *not* mean that the student should pull the head up and elongate the neck. This mistake became popular due to a misinterpretation of the traditional instruction, and shows how mistakes often occur when method and results are confused. Notice the instruction says nothing about the spine. See the section on the spine's shape for a more detailed discussion.

2. Bend your knees

Simply bend your knees a little. Lowering the posture too much is not necessary. With some practice, and when you have some awareness of the Dantian, it is better to think of lowering the body by leading with the centre, rather than just bending the knees.

3. Lift the left heel

Shift the weight to the right leg, balance, and lift the left heel, keeping toes lightly touching the ground, just for balance. If you've been practicing for a while, or if you already have good hip control, be mindful of not tilting the hip sideways when shifting weight.

4. Step shoulder width apart

Place your left foot shoulder-width apart from your right foot. Separating your feet more than shoulder width is not necessary. Some Kungfu styles have the feet further apart, but this is not the case in this particular exercise. It is possible to do so, there are pictures of Chen Xiaowang demonstrating it this way, and I have seen Masters practicing on a wide stance sporadically - but everyday practice is done with the feet only shoulder width apart, or at most a couple of inches wider. If the feet are wider than the shoulders themselves, the posture needs to be a little lower for proportionality.

5. Close your eyes. Body adjustments:
This is the mental procedure to guide you on how to practice:

a. ***Relax your spine, vertebra by vertebra, from top to bottom. Relax your chest. Relax the Dantian. Chest gets empty and Dantian becomes full.***
This aims to bring the body in accordance with Yin and Yang in its upper and lower areas. Students are faced with a conflict between what is natural according to the Dao, and what is considered good by current aesthetic standards. Movies, magazines, superheroes, all exhibit a swollen chest and a sucked in abdomen as signs of virility and strength. This is harmful to one's health, as it accumulates heavy energy in the upper torso. Study the pictures of Chen Xiaowang and Chen Yingjun, you will see how relaxed and empty their chest is, and how full and strong the Dantian area is.

b. ***Shoulders, relax and open. Hips, relax and open. Shoulders and hips flow together and connect.***
The next two instructions and this one are called Three External Harmonies, or Waisanhe. Creating these harmonies is the main goal of Zhanzhuang practice for quite some time. Relaxing means relaxing without changing the posture. Shoulders are a good example: if they are too relaxed, they may "fall" forward, overstretching the muscles in the back, which then sag. It is therefore necessary to relax the shoulders while keeping their correct positioning. Depending on your body and your history, and also your job, it can be quite difficult - for example, if you need to push too hard with the anterior muscles in the shoulder at work, they may be dislocated forward due to over-tensioning of these muscles. It may be that the posterior muscles be lax, or be stiff to compensate for the tension of the anterior muscles. What then? The job of a competent teacher includes positioning your joints as well as possible for you, and guiding you through the gradual process of regaining mobility and well distributed

tone. It is not possible to voluntarily and completely control this: wishing to position or move your shoulders well is not enough, you have to *learn* how to do it. The best way is to try and relax, while keeping the position where the teacher has placed them. This example regards shoulders only - imagine now that every joint in your body needs to go through a similar process to a greater or lesser degree. What does it mean to "relax and open", and what does "flow together and connect" mean? Relaxing and opening is a rough translation of the Chinese expression Fansong. After the first step in relaxation, one which is achieved immediately, from the simple mental command, it is possible to willfully influence a muscle, or the whole joint, in reaching a deeper degree of relaxation. The degree to which one can relax increases with time. We have the illusion we know how to relax, only because the body responds to the mental command as soon as we issue it, but relaxation is a skill, which, like any other, can be extended and developed. Just as you wouldn't walk into a gym expecting to lift a 150kg barbel before a good amount of time in training, you can't expect to relax deeply before a good amount of time in practice. Only when deeper relaxation is achieved, something we call "opening" happens in the joints. Qi trapped in them is released, and, if properly directed, connects with its counterpart in the corresponding joint, according to Waisanhe. This seems all too metaphorical before it happens. After some concrete progress is achieved, you will realize that an actual physical process takes place in your body.

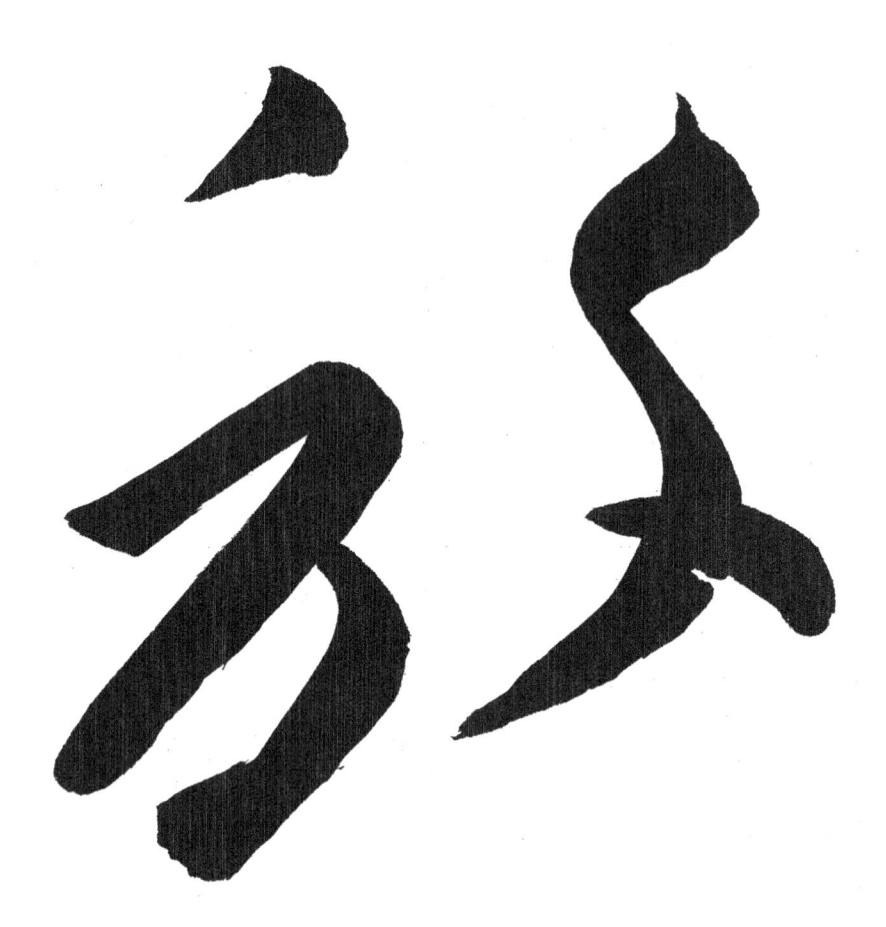

Fàngsōng (放鬆): relax, let oneself go. From fàng 放, release, let go, and sōng 鬆, relax, let go, loosen up.

鬆

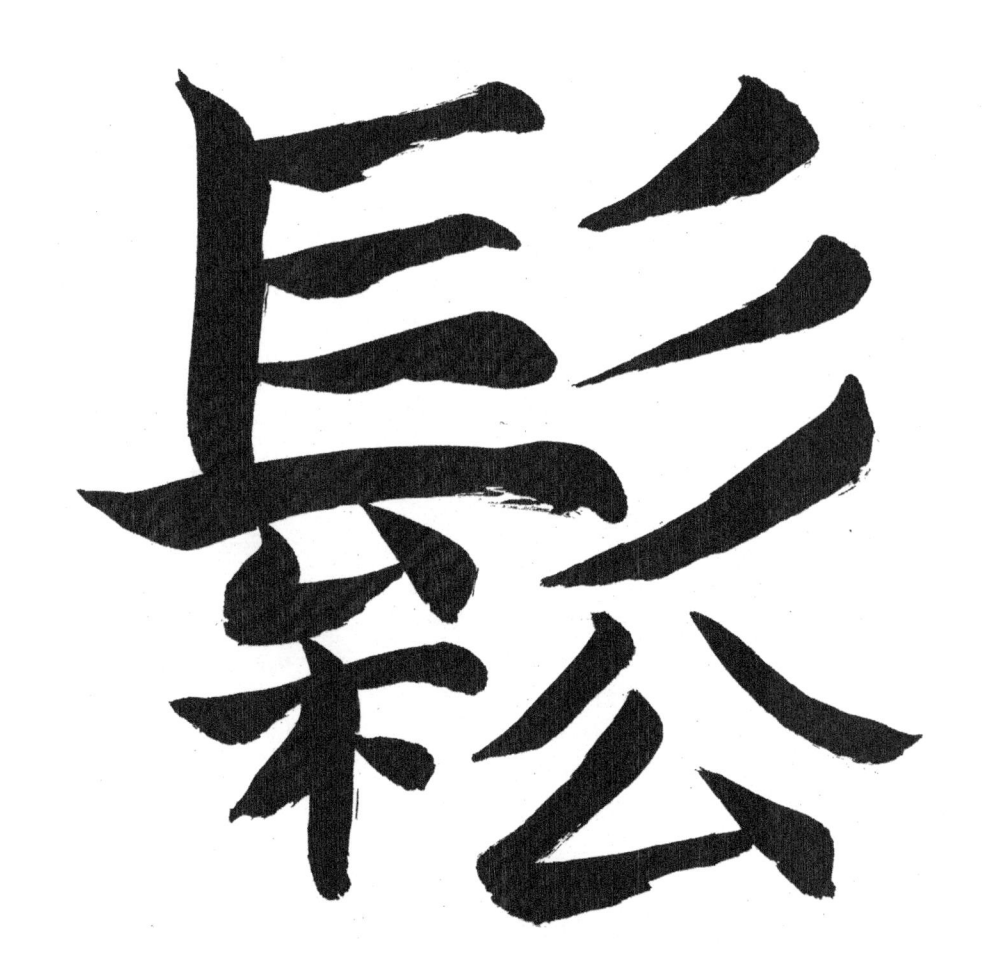

c. *Elbows, relax and open. Knees, relax and open. Elbows and knees flow together and connect.*

d. *Hands, relax and open. Feet, relax and open. Hands and feet flow together and connect.*

e. *The whole body relaxes.*

f. *Slowly raise hands.*
   Arms and hands should be relaxed and light. There should be no weight or force being purposefully exerted. Do not do anything like imagining you are holding or embracing something.

g. *Relax your mind.*
   Do not interfere too much with natural mental processes. Relax and forget.

h. *Listen behind you.*
   Listen behind you, as if you were hearing something a little behind the back of your head. If you are in a perfect place as I described before, it would be ideal to have a stream about 100 metres behind you, and listen to the pleasant, low sound of running water. The reason for listening behind is simple: it is a subterfuge to divert your attention from everyday problems to a place where there is nothing. It also helps to keep your body upright and avoid leaning forward when you start to tire up.

HOW TO END ZHANZHUANG

There is also a prescribed way to end the exercise. Two essential pieces of information are contained in the prescription: first, after half an hour or more of static meditation, it is recommended to slowly and gradually return to the outer world and to movement. Second, we use the state of great introspection we obtained in meditation to start practicing coordinated spiral movement in all joints. The steps to end Zhanzhuang practice are as follows:

1. Slowly lower your hands.
You can take up to a whole minute doing this. It is important not to drop the arms suddenly, letting them fall down, and rather lower them while keeping the internal structure achieved in Zhanzhuang.

2. Cover the Dantian.
Men should have the left palm underneath the right one, touching the abdomen just below the navel. Women should have the right palm underneath the left one. This is a traditional instruction, which we preserve mainly for cultural reasons. Which palm is underneath has no concrete influence on the result.

3. Start Dantian rotation.
Men will first have the hands rotating counterclockwise (from the point of view of someone looking at them from the front), and then in the opposite direction. Women follow the reverse order, according to the same traditional instruction. One performs 36 turns in each direction, if they have practiced Zhanzhuang for half an hour. The number 36 has auspicious meanings in Chinese numerology, but you can do 35 or 40 turns if you prefer. Anything around 40 rotations each way is proportional to thirty minutes of standing. Dantian rotation is an easy exercise because it is simple. However, it is at the same time a difficult one because the movements are smaller. One must see it to understand how to do it, there are no drawings useful enough. The hands' rotation should be done in the plane of one's stomach, and one should take care not to try moving the hips in circles on the floor plane; tilting the body; moving the body only, while keeping the hands static; or varying one's stance height.

4. Bring your hands back to the centre, on the Dantian.

5. Think this: energy flows from the Dantian to your thighs, legs, and feet.
Energy flows from the Dantian to your torso, arms, and hands.
Energy flows from the Dantian to the whole body.

6. Slowly lower your hands.

7. Bring your feet together. Stretch your legs.
Do this slowly. You can reverse the order of these two actions, and one should reverse the order if they have knee problems.

8. Slowly open your eyes, and slowly turn your sight to the outside.

Students often feel lost during Zhanzhuang practice, and do not know what to do while standing still for the 30 minutes this exercise lasts. All you should do is to stand still in the posture where the teacher left you, after adjusting it. It seems little, but it is hard enough to surprise you. Usually the student feels that the teacher is making them lean forward or backwards, and has the feeling that they may even be off balance. The teacher is actually getting the student's body vertical and aligned, but the internal "vertical" reference the student has is based on the incorrect posture they are used to. We are used to thinking we have five senses, but they are actually six. The sixth sense is called proprioception, a word meaning "sense of self," and refers to your body's sense of position. If you work in an environment that has a certain smell, you tend to become insensitive to it. Similarly, if you work leaning forward (for example), you tend to become insensitive to the leaning, and your body gets used to your everyday posture. Your body has, in its joints, specialized neurons that sense joint position and the force exerted by muscles around it. They are true position sensors in the joints, and these sensors can become biased. They end up having their "neutral point" changed in the direction of the everyday posture one adopts.

The student should: keep eyes closed, not move even a millimetre from the position where the teacher places them, and try and relax the whole body while keeping this precise posture. In time, and by repeatedly getting corrections, the student gradually modifies their own body's internal position reference. It is very important to understand that keeping the posture comes first, and relaxing the body comes second. If you relax to the point of moving out of posture, you are relaxing too much. One must know that there are limits to the adjustments a teacher can offer. The most obvious is the teacher's skill - there is no way to teach beyond what one knows. A teacher can only correct a student's posture as well as they can adjust their own posture. The second limit is the student's body, for there are corrections a student may not be able to follow, however simple or small. They may be beyond their body's capacity for relaxation or strength. The third limit is didactic: even if a teacher is skilled, even within the possibilities of the student's body, correcting a student as well as possible is not always productive for learning. If the adjustments are too precise for a student, they might be able to keep the posture or the internal connections for just a few seconds, or an excessive amount of adjustments might be needed, which would cause mental confusion. A student might come to class once every semester and almost always practices alone, in which case the teacher may have to choose the most important adjustments for the student to remember.

After some months in practice, a beginner may experience a variety of misleading sensations. They may get the impression that the posture is unstable after the teacher's corrections, and that the slightest carelessness results in losing the adjustments, and that it is not possible to return to the correct posture no matter how hard they try. This requires more detailed explanation: it is natural that the student initially perceives the correct posture as unstable. The reference for stability in most people is based on locking the joints through muscle tension - which can be done by bringing a joint to the end of its course, or by tensing a combination of muscles and preventing it from moving. In the correct posture for practicing Taijiquan, however, all joints, and especially the hip joints, are in a position where they have the greatest possible freedom of movement. They are loose, never locked, and it is starting from this loose and free posture that the body's integral, connected strength is developed. Students, however, lack strength in their internal connections during the first years of practice, hence the feeling of instability, which can only be overcome over time. If practice is diligent, it will be replaced by a feeling of simultaneous stability and mobility. What about not being able to return to the correct posture, if one deviates from it? As we said, a student does not have enough internal power during the first years in learning. Reaching the correct posture on their own is not possible, because they simply don't have enough strength to align the joints as required, moreover they don't know exactly where the alignment is. It sounds like a hopeless situation, but helping overcome it is a teacher's job: getting the student's body into the correct posture, so they develop strength and cultivate an internal reference for the correct alignment. We must emphasize the student's part is relaxing the whole body, without any exceptions, while keeping the posture without moving.

Afterwards, the student may feel these sensations tend to repeat in cycles, with progressively less intensity. Strength and accuracy of the internal alignments reference gradually increase, and the student will feel their ability to relax, even under effort, increases at the same time, and the more they relax, the more strength is needed to keep the posture. Tendons, ligaments and muscles will naturally stretch during the process. It is important to remember strength and relaxation are closely linked and are not mutually exclusive - on the contrary, strength is needed in order to relax. Imagine yourself supporting a load greater than you are capable of: your whole body will inevitably tense up. On the other hand, if the load is very small, it will be easy to bear it with a relaxed body. It happens that in a correct posture, with good internal alignments, the demand on the muscles is very intense. It will take years long training to be able to keep the correct posture while simultaneously relaxing. Relaxation, if cultivated in a good posture, generates power: remember that power and relaxation are a Yin-Yang pair.

How to distribute weight on the feet is a common question. Weight should be equally divided on both feet - but this is too general an instruction. After the teacher adjusts your posture, you may in fact feel more weight on one foot, or more work on one leg than the other. This may be due to your body not having the same strength on both sides, or on both legs. When the teacher places you in the centre, you will feel the weaker side working harder, causing the impression that there is more "weight" on it. The same advice mentioned before applies: keep the posture in which your teacher has set you. There is also the question of how to distribute the weight on the soles of each feet. Weight should be equally distributed on the entire sole, but again I caution, this is a general instruction, as the feeling of where the weight is can change over time. In the first few months or years, the weight usually seems to be somewhat towards the heels, later on it seems to be more towards the front of the feet. What you should keep in mind is the weight is distributed over the entire sole.

A very important process called "Distinguishing Yin and Yang" takes place during Taijiquan learning. As we've seen, Yin and Yang are inseparable. We figuratively say that Yin and Yang are in a chaotic state, or disorderly mixed, in an untrained individual. This is a somewhat exaggerated interpretation, as the physiological processes are occurring normally: the heart is beating, lungs are breathing, organs are functioning as they should. They may be more, or less well regulated, maybe disturbed by the stress of daily rush, but they are in general fulfilling their duties. There is nevertheless a fair degree of disorder, especially in posture, movement, and refined mental processes, which we abbreviate here with the word chaos. The standing posture in Zhanzhuang is often called Wuji posture. Wuji is an undifferentiated state, when Yin and Yang are not yet separated. The name Wuji Posture for the Zhanzhuang exercise is also a figurative name, since Zhanzhuang is the first step in distinguishing Yin and Yang in your body. Even though it is a static and symmetrical exercise; even though it can, in its more advanced stages, be a path to bringing the student to experience Emptiness, we are still in the manifest world, subject to duality. Understanding what to do is much easier in Zhanzhuang because the posture is technically simple enough. Upper body (from the waist up) belongs to Yang, and lower body belongs to Yin, so the upper body should be empty and light, and the lower body should be full and heavy. This is reflected in the instructions by the sentence "chest becomes empty and Dantian fills up". During practice, the feeling is one's weight is going down to the feet, and you feel them pressing harder and harder against the ground. The feet can even develop a burning feeling. It is also very usual for the thighs to burn; sometimes, or for periods that may last a few months, the student may feel tremors in the legs and hips, from intense exertion. Feet, calves and thighs burn because they are not used to supporting the full weight of the body. We remove undue loads from tendons and ligaments, and place them on the large muscles, transmitting them without fraying or overloading the joints. It is necessary to warn the reader that fatigue, trembling and burning, are transient sensations - they may persist for a long time, until enough strength naturally develops, but they are only consequences of physical work, they are not expressions of the principle governing practice. Do not try to get the weight of the body on your thighs in order to get a sensation of exercising, or of burning legs. Weight should go to the soles of your feet - if you try to feel your thighs burning, the energy will be blocked at knee height. The power your legs develop should be natural. Another important warning is about the difference between feeling large muscles burn, and feeling sharp pain. Burning is one thing, and pain is a completely different one: there can be no pain, and in particular no joint pain. Often the word "pain" is used in place of "burning", sometimes even Taijiquan Masters make this exchange - but we must never confuse pain resulting from a blockage with burning resulting from load on a muscle. There are exceptions, but they are very rare and require personalized guidance. Pain means an impediment in the circulation of Qi, and you should immediately inform the teacher if you feel pain, so they can analyze your posture and adjust it. Big muscles may burn, but the joints cannot hurt.

If the upper body is not empty, that is, if the body is not light above the waist, you are making the much talked about mistake of Double Weight, or Double Yin. Feet will always be heavy, because you are standing. If your chest is heavy, you have heavy top and bottom, violating distribution of Yin and Yang according to the order of Dao. Or, to put it another way, you are going against the law of gravity. The Double Weight mistake can manifest itself in various ways in the body, in many degrees of different subtlety. Continued progress in practice involves, in one sense, distinguishing Yin and Yang in ever more refined ways. This is not unlike what the texts about meditation and Zen tell us. The allegory of agitated muddy water is well known: if you have muddy water, and you let it stand still (for example in a calm lake, or in a container), mud separates from the water and settles to the bottom as movement decreases. Zhanzhuang causes precisely this to happen. In Taijiquan, we start with the body. This, incidentally, exposes the process by which one can attain the state of meditation by practicing Zhanzhuang. Practice can be more physical or more meditative according to each person, in the first months or years, but Zhanzhuang always offers a significant calming effect. As the student becomes familiar with it, the coarser part of energy descends and concentrates in the lower part of the body; the more skill improves, the less Yin energy remains at the top, and gradually the mind starts to perceive emptiness and silence. When the top is emptied, nothing remains. This is meditation, achieved naturally.

With even more practice, it is possible to realize the energy goes up on the body's back (Yang), and goes down on its front (Yin). It is not necessary to do anything for it to happen, rather, there is actually nothing to be done. Just practice according to the principles, and this will be the natural result. There is no "key" or secret. It is not possible to force this state or its perceiving, and if the student tries to do so, they may suffer undesirable effects such as headaches and tension. From now on, perseverance is no longer the motivation for daily practice. The body asks for practice, and you miss it greatly when some unforeseen event steals your personal practice time. After some more time, it is possible to come to feel that within Yang, Yin is born, and within Yin, Yang is born: at the same time that energy flows up the back, there is also a more subtle descent of energy through the back; at the same time the energy descends on the front of the body, there is also a more subtle ascent of energy on the front. This is an effect of Daoist Alchemy, obtained naturally, that is, following the method of Dao itself.

Zhanzhuang changes your body. You're not simply trying to learn a technique, not just strengthening your body or your legs, not just meditating, not just doing an isometric exercise. You are trying to *transform* your body. This is an idea coming from Daoism, that it is possible to transmute one's body. Your body's shape will change, relationships between muscles, how you distribute power within it and how you stand will change, and you will develop a completely new motor coordination. The integration of your mind and your body will be strengthened and have a new meaning. You are trying to transform your body so that Waisanhe is its natural state.

Chansigong

Silk Reeling is the Qigong that summarizes everything we're trying to do in Taijiquan. In a seminar with Grandmaster Chen Xiaowang in Brazil, a friend of mine asked him: what's the purpose of this exercise, what are we trying to learn here? Chen Xiaowang replied: if you learn this, you will have learned Taijiquan. His words must not be taken lightly. I was once staying at the same house where he was hosted, and at the age of 60, after more than fifty years practicing, he kept doing Chansigong every morning.

Silk Reeling is the perfect name for this Qigong, and it wasn't chosen only for its poetic beauty. Most importantly, the movement is performed in spirals. At first glance, one's hands appear to describe circles, and one must stay mindful of the movement being made of spirals and not simple circles. In a spiral, there is a component of entry or exit in relation to the centre, and in this exercise Qi goes out and comes in cyclically. Like when unwinding a cocoon's silk thread, there is an exact amount of force needed to accomplish the movement. Teachers almost always tell students to "relax", at the same time adjusting the student's posture. This is actually the most didactic and productive teaching method, and it is also the best way forward for the student: they should seek to copy the form (posture, appearance, fluidity and movement), while at the same time trying to relax. The effect, if the didactic is diligently followed by the student, is causing the body to generate a precise amount of physical strength. In technical terms, we say there is a precise amount of tension to perform the movement, which is right in the middle between excessive tension and excessive relaxation. Think about it: if someone practicing Taijiquan really relaxed, they would fall on the ground and lay there, motionless. What we call relaxation is different from common sense understanding, it's the Middle Way between tense and flaccid. When unwinding silk from a cocoon, if you apply too much force, the silk thread will be broken; if you apply too little force, the thread will become entangled. The same happens here.

Chen Xiaowang created Chansigong, but he didn't come up with it out of nowhere. He looked in the Forms for the simplest moves, the ones most representative of Taijiquan's fundamental skills, and presented them in a repetitive fashion, creating didactics adapted for present times. You could say that Taijiquan forms are long Silk Reeling exercises. It wouldn't be a complete description, but you wouldn't be wrong. One could in principle choose any movement in the form, and practice it repeatedly like Chansigong; good examples would be Hands Making Circles and Three Steps Forward. According to Chen Xiaowang's didactics, there are 19 Silk Reeling exercises, divided into two groups of 10 and 9 exercises respectively. Exercises in the first group are simpler, and recommended for the first years of learning. Exercises in the second group are much more difficult, requiring a degree of stability and postural structure that a beginner does not have. We often teach the exercises in the second group even to beginners, because it is interesting they at least know the exercises. Knowing and hearing the explanations about them creates a more complete picture of the movement system, which helps learning. On the other hand, I seldom teach exercises in the second group during class. Chen Yingjun used to say that until skill is at reasonable level, practicing the second group exercises regularly would not be productive. Nineteen exercises may seem daunting, but there are actually not that many. In the first group, if we adopt a more optimistic outlook, there are only three, not ten exercises: one-handed, two-handed, and backing up. The first two are done on both sides, on a fixed stance and while stepping, and the last one is done on two sides - this is why we count ten variations. One could say in the second group there are actually four exercises, and their variations.

We now need to get into the more technical aspects of movement, so we need to think about the space where the body moves. Please stand (or imagine yourself) in a room, facing one of the walls. We need three planes to describe movement: the wall in front of you is the Coronal plane, the wall by your side represents the Sagittal plane, and the floor represents the Transverse plane. Grandmaster Chen Xiaowang described the Dantian's movement using only *two* planes. He says the phrase "One Principle, Three Techniques" when referring to this way of describing movement. The Principle he refers to is the Centre Moves and Hand Follows. Three Techniques are: moving the Dantian in the Coronal plane, moving the Dantian in the Sagittal plane, and the mixture of these two movements. In reality, almost all movements in the Taijiquan Form use the Third Technique - but this would be too complicated to learn. Therefore, in the first several years of practice, what one should do is try and learn the First Technique, and practice the Form looking for it. With time and gradual progress of skill and strength, the student will begin to notice, first in simpler movements, then in more complex ones, how the Second Technique is mixed with the First.

Why would Chen Xiaowang explain the Dantian's movement using only two planes, the Sagittal and the Coronal ones? Why wouldn't he talk about the movement in the Transverse plane? After all, shouldn't we rotate our body around the vertical axis, or the spine? Answering these questions requires a mathematical explanation, but we can replace it with a practical demonstration. We will show, by means of figures, that it is unnecessary to speak of movement in the Transverse plane (or turning the body around a vertical axis, which is the same). You will see that if you take any object and move it in the Coronal plane and then in the Sagittal plane, you will have also movement in the Transverse plane as an obligatory result. Take this chair, for example:

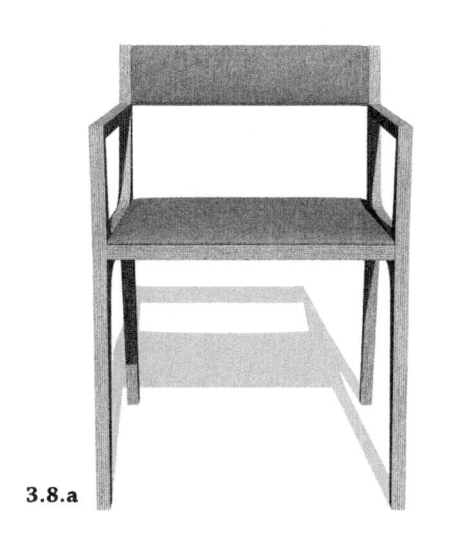

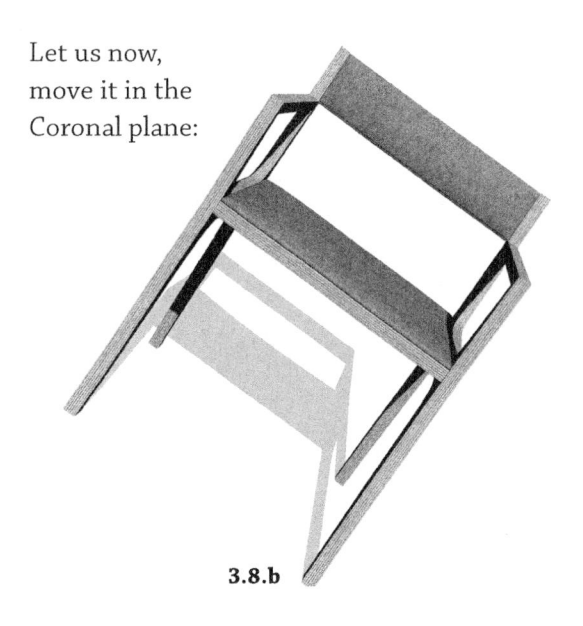

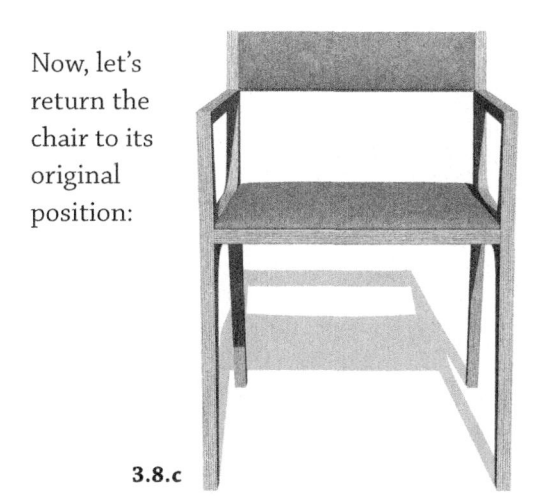

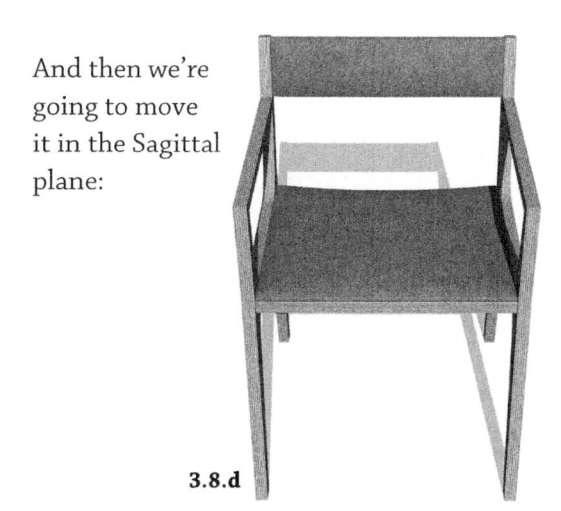

Let us now, move it in the Coronal plane:

3.8.a

3.8.b

Now, let's return the chair to its original position:

And then we're going to move it in the Sagittal plane:

3.8.c

3.8.d

Trivial, right? Now I will get the chair back to the original position:

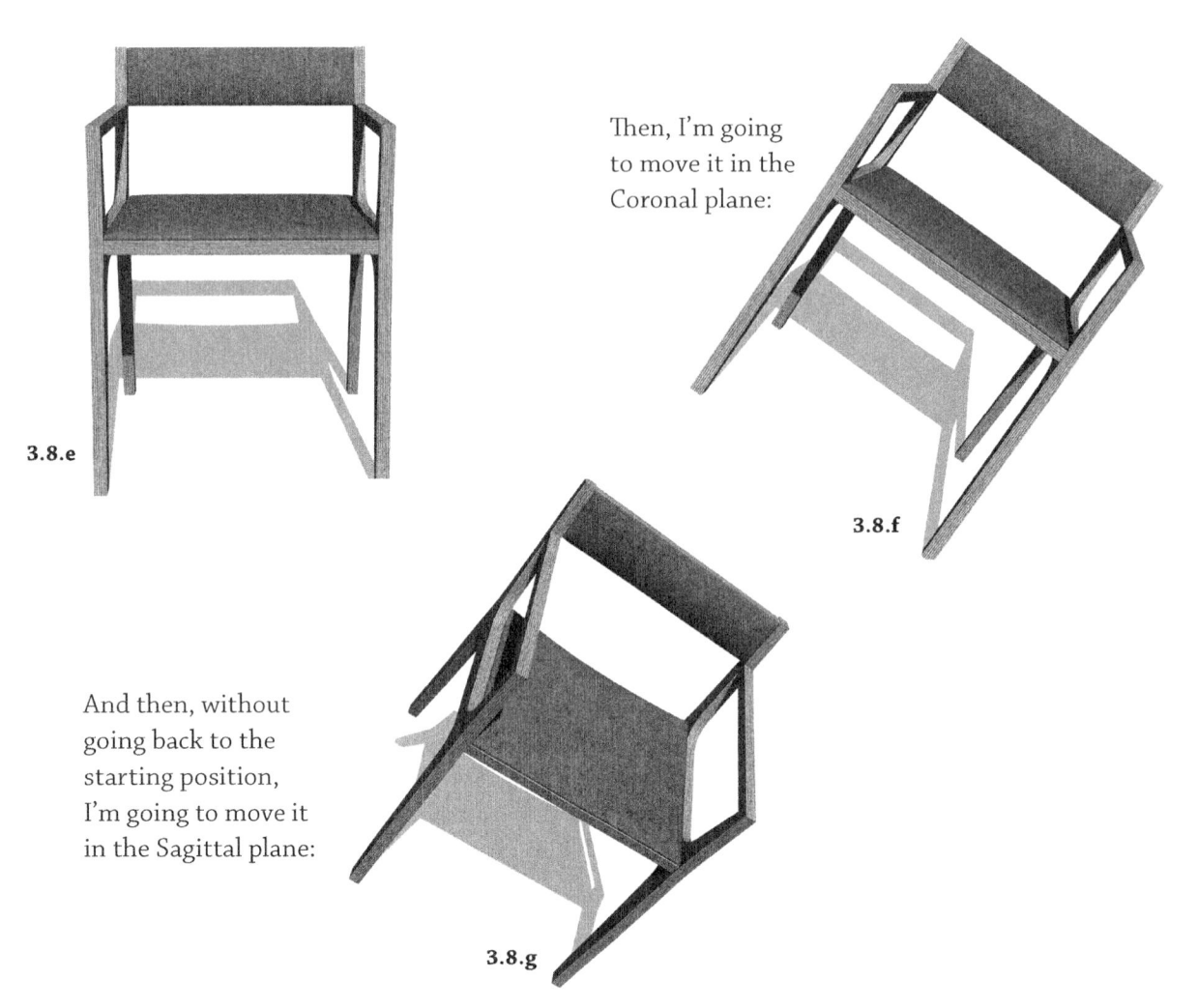

Then, I'm going to move it in the Coronal plane:

3.8.e

3.8.f

And then, without going back to the starting position, I'm going to move it in the Sagittal plane:

3.8.g

Notice the chair is a little sideways, as you can now see its side. The consequence of moving it in the Coronal and Sagittal planes was it ended up changing direction: a movement also happened in the Transverse plane. This is inevitable, it is a mathematical necessity, it is a property of the three-dimensional space in which we live. The same phenomenon happens with your body's centre, it is the reason you end up turning around your vertical axis and slightly changing the direction you face during Chansigong. However, you should not try to turn your body to the side in this exercise. Slightly changing direction must be a consequence of simultaneous Dantian movement in the Coronal and Sagittal planes.

The explanation offered by Grandmaster Chen Xiaowang is nothing short of genius. He was able to explain in a simple way how the body should move if subjected to the constraining conditions of Waisanhe. When you are able to feel what Chen Xiaowang has put into words, you will realize there could be no more economical, elegant and clearer way of describing movement. We could say that if the body is connected as required by Waisanhe, there are only three things you can do with it: coil it, fold it, or a mixture of these two. This is the same as Chen Xiaowang has said more clearly and precisely. Incidentally, the verbs I used in the above sentence are important. When teaching in English, Masters usually choose the phrase *turn body*. The verb "turn", however, may give the impression that all you need to do is turn your hips to the side. That is not what you should try to do, or at the very least is not all you should try to do after you have some experience in practice. The Chinese character in the texts would be better translated as coil. On the other hand, the verb coil would bring along other problems and complications too big to be dealt with in a group class. I believe this is why the Grandmaster chose *turn* instead of *coil*. The body is slightly and naturally coiled as it follows the Dantian, without it being done forcibly. An analogous complication arises with the verb fold. When the Dantian moves in the Sagittal plane, the whole body gently folds and unfolds, and the Grandmaster calls this "folding method" in his instructional videos. However, it is not enough to simply flex the joints.

YIN AND YANG IN MOTION

When we leave a static posture, as exemplified by Zhanzhuang, and start moving, Yin and Yang become more evident. In Zhanzhuang, the most apparent characteristics of the interaction between Yin and Yang are opposition and complementarity. In Chansigong, alternation and mutual generation become visible. In order to analyze these properties, we need to take into account the passing of time. Let's use the seasons as an example: spring, summer, fall, and winter. Which two are the most Yang? In which are expansion and warmth more evident? Clearly, in spring and summer - but between these two, which one shows Yang more completely? We can see that in four seasons, two of them are more Yang and two more Yin, and among the more

Yang, we see one where Yang is emerging, and another where Yang is complete; among the more Yin, we see one where Yin is in its youth, and another where Yin is mature.

The Yi Jing (I Ching - Classic of Changes) represents Yang by a whole, strong line, and Yin by a broken one.

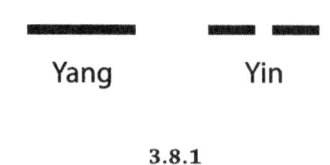

Yang   Yin

3.8.1

Arranging these representations next to the Taiji diagram, we have

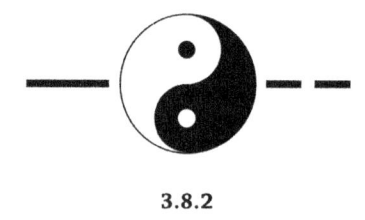

3.8.2

If we want to represent four states of alternating Yin and Yang, as in the passing of the four seasons described above, we need two lines, as in the figure below. In the Yi Jing, the following images are called Four Appearances of Yin and Yang.

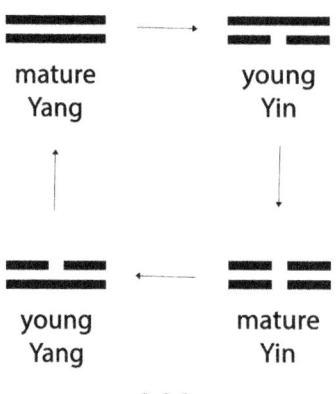

mature Yang   young Yin

young Yang   mature Yin

3.8.3

The Four Appearances, being an unfolding of Yin and Yang, can be used to analyze many natural phenomena, with more resolution. If we take day and night, day is more Yang, and night is more Yin. If we use the Four Appearances, sunrise is Young Yang (the starting Yang), noon is Mature Yang (the complete Yang), sunset is Young Yin, and midnight is Mature Yin. When the day reaches noon, we are at the maximum of Yang, and from then on Yin begins to increase, until it becomes visible at sunset: when one of them (in this case the Yang) reaches its extreme, it begets its opposite. We call this Mutual Generation. The same happens at midnight: from then on, when Yin has reached its maximum, Yang is born within Yin.

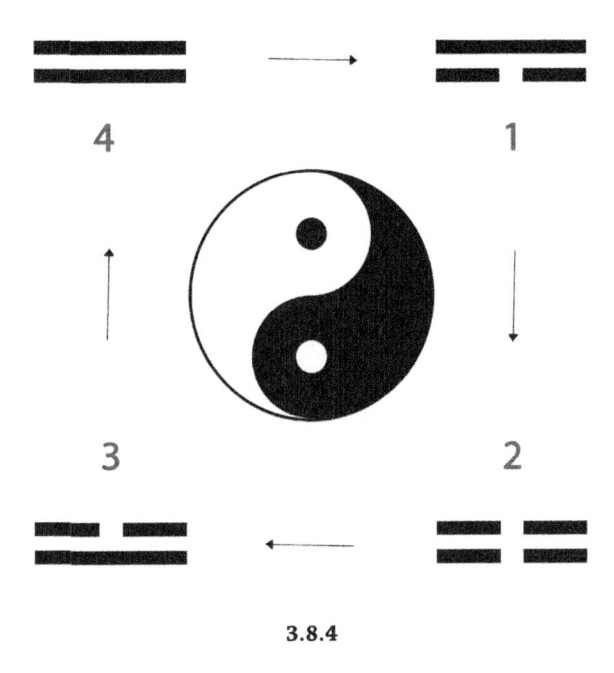

3.8.4

This is shown in the Yin-Yang diagram by the black dot within the large white area, and the white dot within the large black area. In the Yi Jing, by convention, progressive changes are shown in the lines from bottom to top. Therefore, by following the arrow from No. 4 to No. 1, one sees Yin appears first in the bottom position, then propagates to the top position, when Yin attains completion in No. 2. Similarly, in No. 3, Yang appears in the bottom position, and in No. 4 propagates to the top position, when Yang attains completion.

DIDACTICS OF SILK REELING

Chen Xiaowang created a series of standardized steps for starting and performing Silk Reeling exercises. They comprise five steps to get to a starting posture, and then four repeating steps of execution. The five steps for starting the exercises are:

1. Keep your head upright, keep your body straight.
2. Bend your knees.
3. Lift your heel (left or right, depending on the side).
4. Step to the side (about one and a half to two shoulder widths).
5. Adopt the initial posture (to adjust to the standardized four step counting).

These are the same steps as for starting Zhanzhuang. When starting Chansigong, you should reach the same inner state of stillness and silence as during standing meditation, and you should be able to create the same internal structure with Waisanhe. It won't be as easy as when standing: you will be moving, making spirals, shifting your weight, with your eyes open.

For simplicity's sake, I'll use the most basic of the Silk Reeling exercises, Frontal Chansigong. I must emphasize what I said about didactic material in the Introduction: the following descriptions are necessarily limited, and apply to a specific stage in Taijiquan's learning process. They should be used as long as they are productive, then they should be discarded.

The four steps in Chansigong are as follows (assuming the right hand moving, as in the accompanying illustrations). Please note, when interpreting right and left, that you are looking frontally at a person and "right" and "left" will seem reversed.

1. In order to perform step 1, first adopt position 4 in Figure 3.8.8. Keep your weight on the right foot, and slightly turn the body right, turning the palm of your hand forward (the fingers will be pointing to the right when you finish).
2. Shift your weight to your left foot while bringing your hand closer to your body, and turn your palm upwards.
3. Keep your weight on your left foot, and turn your body left, raising your forearm to shoulder height, and turning your palm downward.
4. Shift your weight to your right foot, turning the palm outward.

The four phases in Chansigong obey the natural waxing and waning of Yin and Yang, and like other natural phenomena, can be described using the Four Appearances.

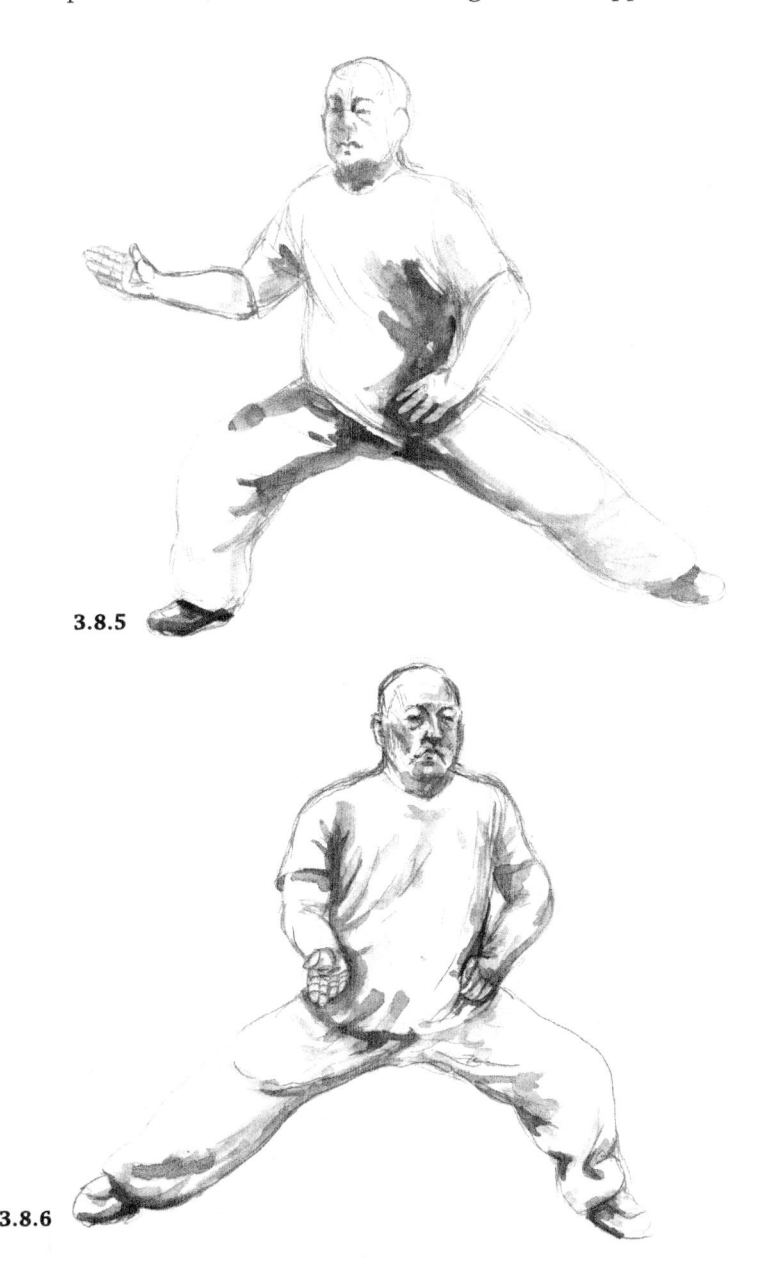

3.8.5

3.8.6

This exercise's choreography is very simple. In one or two months, taking one or two classes a week, most people are ready to try practicing by themselves at home.

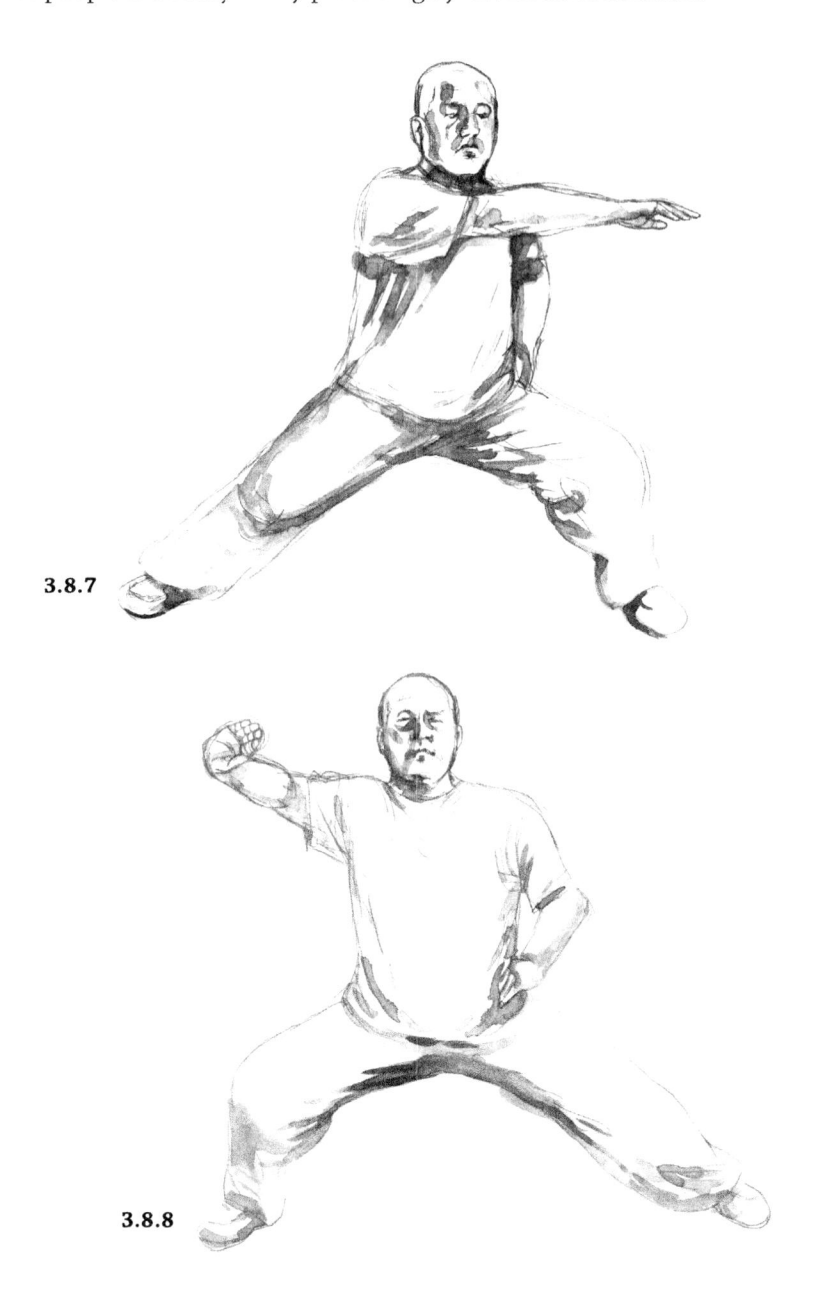

3.8.7

3.8.8

Please notice that in steps 1 and 3 the body is turning, and in steps 2 and 4 the weight is shifting from one foot to the other.

At first, it's necessary to distinguish very clearly between Yin and Yang. In each phase of the exercise, there's a change, and we can look at the changes themselves from the viewpoint of Yin and Yang. In phases 1 and 3 a change in the quality of energy is taking place. Before phase 1, energy had been expanding, and after phase 1, it is retracting; therefore, in phase 1 there is a transformation from Yang to Yin. Before phase 3 energy was collecting towards the centre, and after phase 3, it is expanding towards the extremity. That's why we say that in phase 3 there is a change from Yin to Yang. In phases 2 and 4 there is no change in quality but rather in quantity: in phase 2 the energy completes its retraction, in phase 4 the energy completes its expansion. We could say that in phases 1 and 3, when there is a change in quality, the transformation is more "internal," therefore more Yin; in phases 2 and 4, when there is a change in quantity, the transformation is more "external," therefore more Yang. In the first months of practice it is necessary to separate very clearly the actions of turning the body and shifting weight: either you turn your body, or you shift the weight. You cannot do both simultaneously, or else you will be less balanced. Please see the following figure on how the exercise should be done.

THE LITTLE TAIJIQUAN MANUAL FOR BEGINNERS

Please notice: from step 1 to step 2, the weight shifts, but the direction the body is facing stays the same. From step 2 to step 3, the body turns, but weight stays in the same place. From step 3 to step 4, the weight shifts sides, but the direction the body faces stays the same. From step 4 to step 1, the body turns, but weight stays in the same place. For most people, practicing this way for some time is absolutely essential. If it is not done, they will not be able to teach their body to

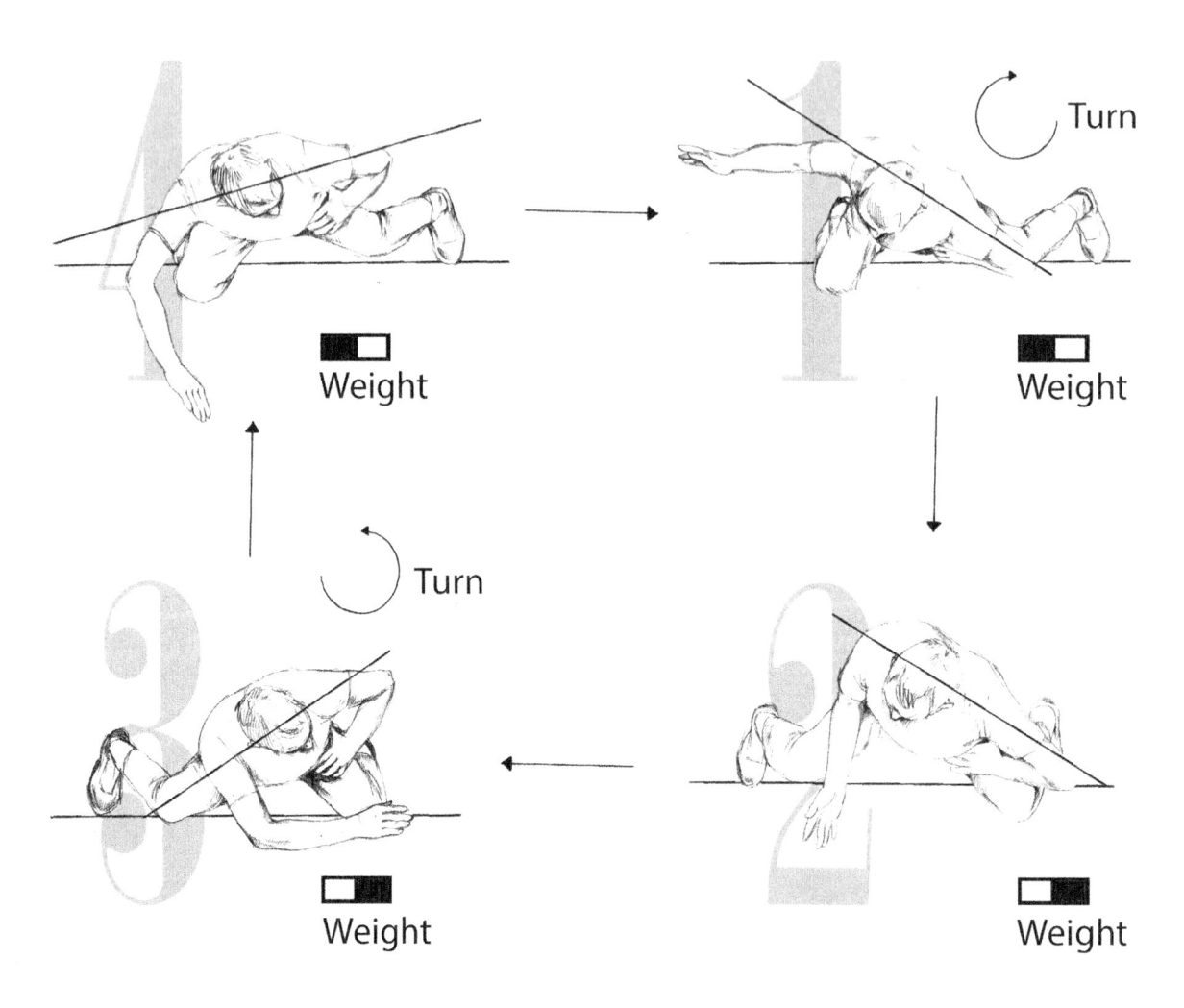

THE LITTLE TAIJIQUAN MANUAL FOR BEGINNERS

differentiate one action from the other, and the desired motor coordination will not be achieved.

After a good while, the beginner spontaneously notices that in positions 2 and 4, the teacher is actually facing forward (as shown in 3.8.6 and 3.8.8), and not slightly diagonal as shown in the previous figure. When they notice it, it is probably time for them to progress to the second stage in learning Chansigong, as shown in the next figure:

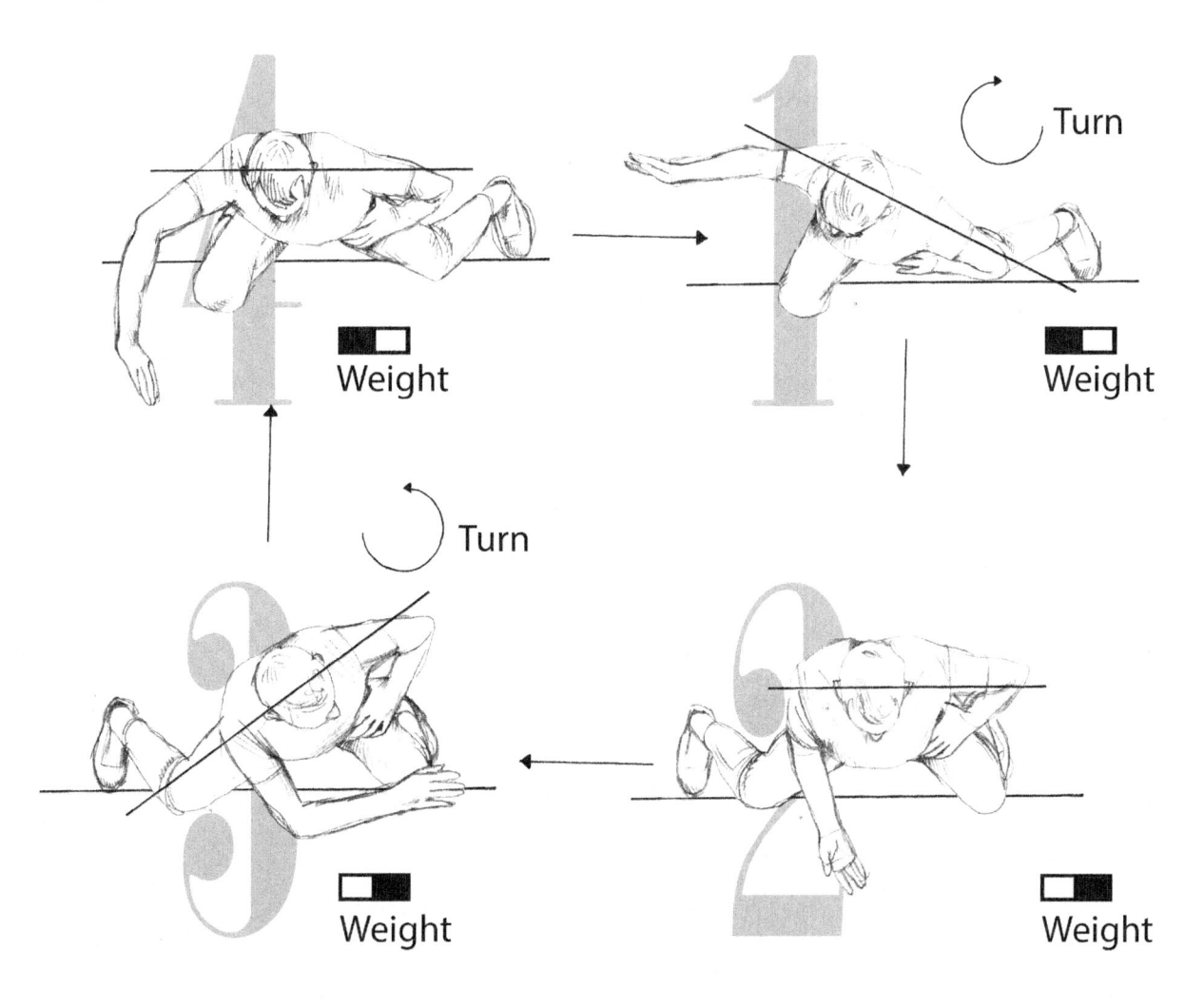

3.8.10

You will notice in phases 2 and 4 there was actually a little turning in the body. This means that after very clearly distinguishing turning from shifting, we can now allow a little interpenetration in them, which is more natural. It is essential that the student understands they should not try to rotate the body in phases 2 and 4. They should just shift their weight sideways, let the body adjust itself, and finish phases 2 and 4 facing forward - that is, with the hip, chest, and shoulders parallel to the reference direction. If they instead try turning while shifting weight, it is nearly certain they will overshoot the reference direction, which is a far worse and more difficult error to correct than not reaching the reference direction.

It's possible to perform any action in Chansigong both in excess and in lacking. It is possible to turn the body too much, and it is also possible to turn it too little. It is possible, when shifting weight, to move too far towards the foot receiving the weight, and it is also possible to move too little. The challenge in learning lies precisely here: finding the Middle Way. Performing actions in excess or in deficiency is in fact very easy, but finding the exact point between the two extremes is very difficult, as the Middle Way changes with countless variables, that in turn change dynamically. Taking one specific learner as an object of observation, let us suppose they use a constant distance between their feet when practicing Chansigong as described here. For this person, there is a personalized ideal posture height - if they stand too high, they will not exercise enough, if they stand too low, they will end up stiffening and will not be able to turn their body comfortably. If they stand too high, it will be difficult judge the weight shift precisely, or they may tend to shift the weight too much and overshoot; if they stand too low, they may not be able to move their body sideways as much as needed because the load on their leg muscles might be too intense. Standing at the ideal height is quite important - the problem is the ideal height varies for every individual student even during a single day, even if they stand with their feet always the same distance apart. The ideal height, if the student practices in the early hours, may be a little higher, until they have warmed up; if they practice at the end of the day, they may be overtired from work, which needs to be taken into account. The ideal amount of any action varies with the weather, the season, the amount of sleep one had the night before, and other factors. As said before: there are no fixed geometric standards. It is told that a Taijiquan Master was once asked, "Master, in such a posture, should the right foot be at 30° or 45°?" The Master would have looked, tested it both ways, and replied, "Son, when I learned this, I didn't even know what a degree was" - which is true, as he must have started practicing before attending school as a child. What the story means is position and alignment should be felt, there is a range of acceptable variation (including for stance height), and strict geometric norms are of little use. One exception of note concerns the reference direction, the direction one is "facing". It is important that, when one finishes phases 2 and 4, they end up facing the reference direction.

The issue of stance height brings our attention to flexibility. The average student has generally less than desirable flexibility. If they go too low in a stance they will not be able to turn their body, on the other hand, if they don't go low enough they will feel nearly nothing. Since strength and flexibility are complementary, there is a trade-off between them: if you use all your flexibility to get to a low stance, you will be stiff.

Qi circulation, during Chansigong, takes place as follows:

1. Qi returns from fingertips down the arm, and then down the body's side to the waist.
2. Qi returns from the waist to Dantian.
3. Qi goes from Dantian to the back, and up the spine to the 7th cervical vertebra.
4. Qi circulates to shoulder, elbow, hand, and fingertips.

This information is useful for long term progress, and to reassure the curious student, who usually has questions on this matter. Its concrete usefulness in the first years, on the other hand, is very limited, and should not be overestimated. It must be stressed that one should not practice Chansigong with it in mind, as it is not the path to learning, rather the result of training. Chen Yingjun is very direct when asked about Qi circulation during his seminars: "It is enough to think about concentrating Qi in the Dantian". This is the same teaching I heard from his father, in a private class in 1999. You must walk the path, not fantasize about the destination. What is the path? First, you must practice as I have just explained in the preceding text. Secondly, your teacher must:

- Skillfully demonstrate the movement so you can copy it.
- Hold your hips with their hands, and move them for you, so you can feel how you should move.
- Hold your arm and hand and move them for you, so you feel can how they connect and move with your body.

Thirdly, you must remember the principles during your practice - most especially, you must remember: the Centre Leads and the Hand Follows.

THE LITTLE TAIJIQUAN MANUAL FOR BEGINNERS

REMARKS ON COMMON MISTAKES

In my teaching experience there are some mistakes that new students tend to show very commonly. This section is a warning for you to try and avoid them, but it is no substitute for receiving careful adjustments from a good teacher. The key to recognizing and correcting your mistakes is reflecting on the application of Taijiquan's principles. See the following picture:

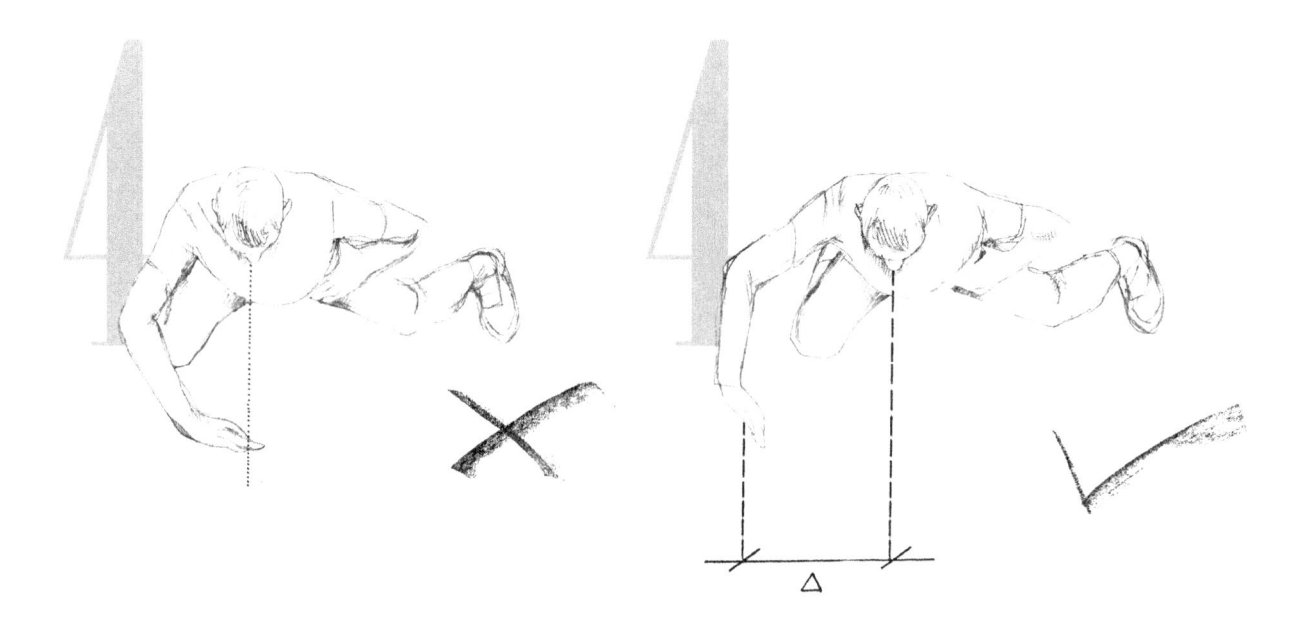

3.8.11

In the leftmost illustration, the student finished phase 4 in Frontal Chansigong, but the hand is still in front of his chest (his palm is facing out, which is correct). Why is this a mistake? Hands follow Dantian. If the Dantian moved sideways during phase 4, the hand must also move sideways - not only because the whole body moved sideways, but the hand itself must move sideways in relation to the body, getting away from the centreline and moving to the side, as the rightmost illustration shows. If this is not done so, Qi will not expand enough to the hand and fingers.

In Chansigong's phase 2, a similar error may happen:

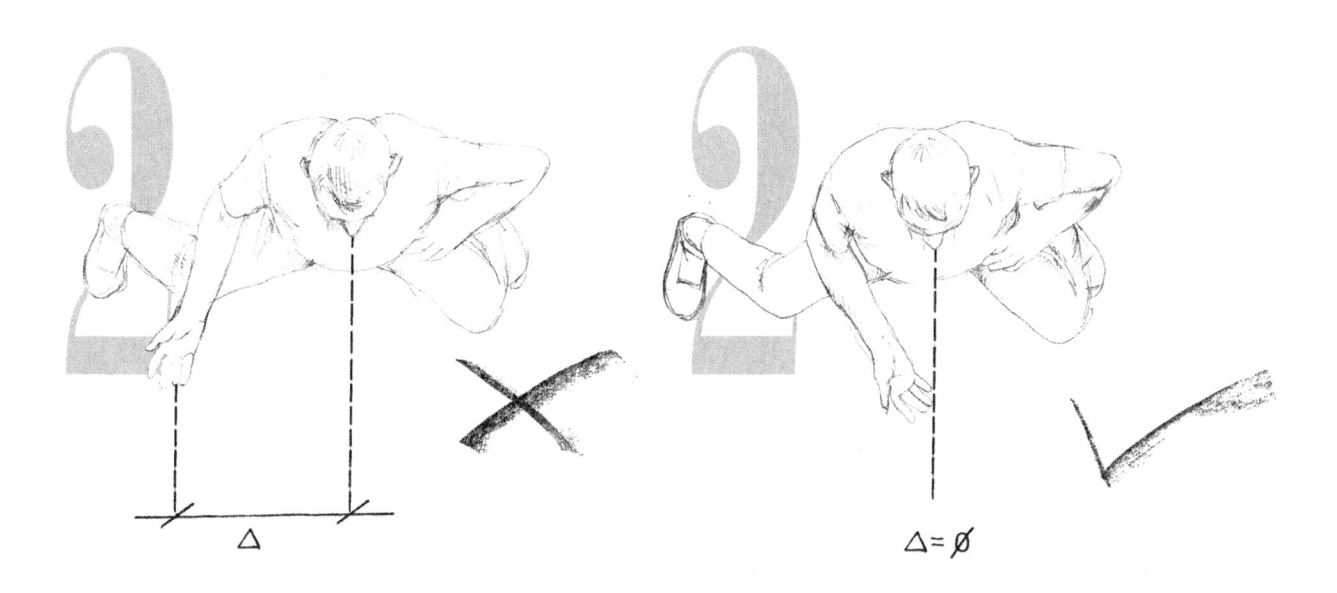

3.8.12

Here, the error occurs when the hand does not return to near the centreline of the body. In this case, Qi doesn't return well to the centre, and the hand becomes heavy, causing the next phase to be difficult.

In phase 3 the most prevalent error is this:

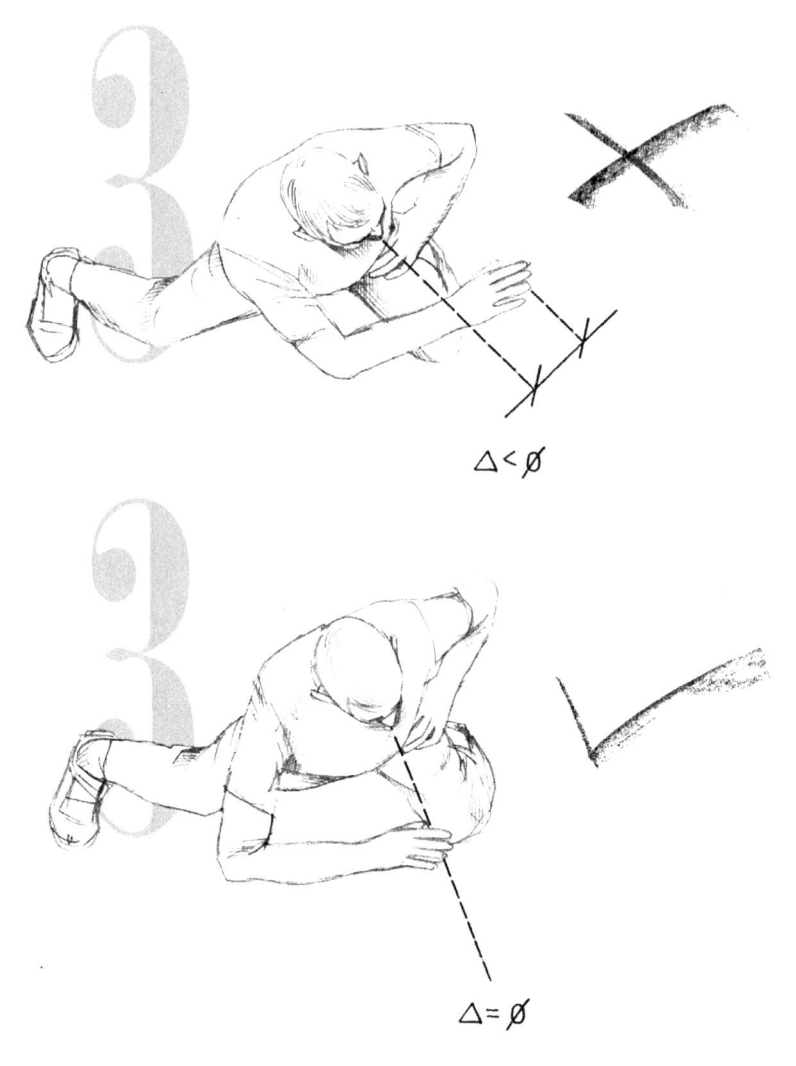

△ < ∅

△ = ∅

3.8.13

THE LITTLE TAIJIQUAN MANUAL FOR BEGINNERS

When rotating the body, the student makes a mistake in moving the hand sideways. At the end of step 2, the hand was near the body's centreline, and from that moment onwards the Dantian turns - but does not move sideways. Therefore, the hand should turn, but not move sideways. When the student moves the hand as shown in the topmost illustration, the shoulder becomes tense and rises.

Why are these errors common? It will now become clear why practicing a slightly "square" version of Chansigong is necessary for some time, as shown in figure 3.8.9. See the following error:

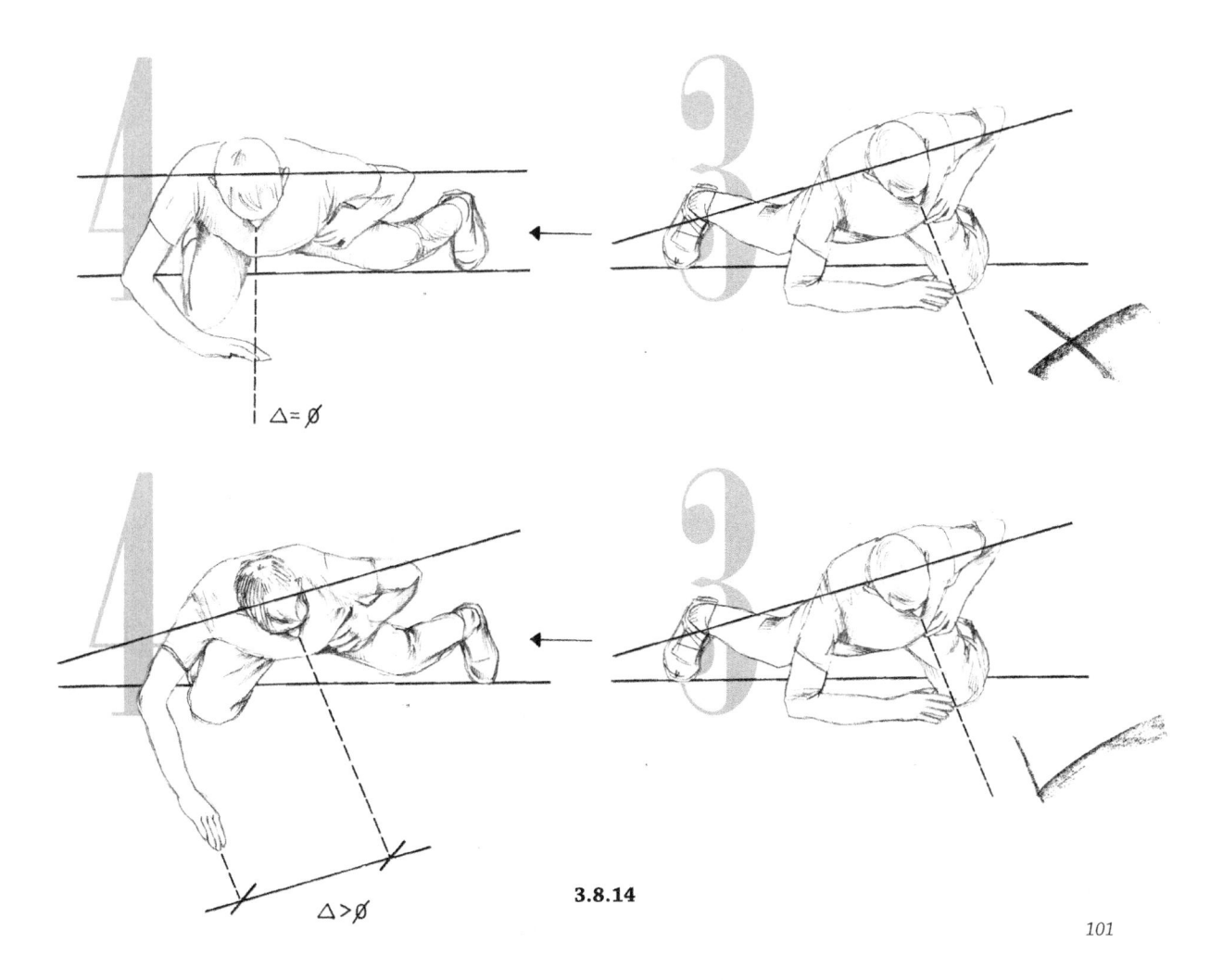

△ = ∅

△ > ∅

3.8.14

101

Here, when performing phase 4, the student confused turning their body with shifting their weight. They tried to turn the body at the same time they moved the body sideways to the right, shifting the weight, and had the mistaken impression that their hand was moved sideways too. This did not happen, the hand stayed in front of the body. The solution is practicing Chansigong while emphatically separating the actions of shifting weight and turning body: when shifting weight, only shift your weight (as in the lower part of the preceding picture), when turning the body, only turn the body.

Here is the same problem, this time in phase 2, and its solution, at the bottom:

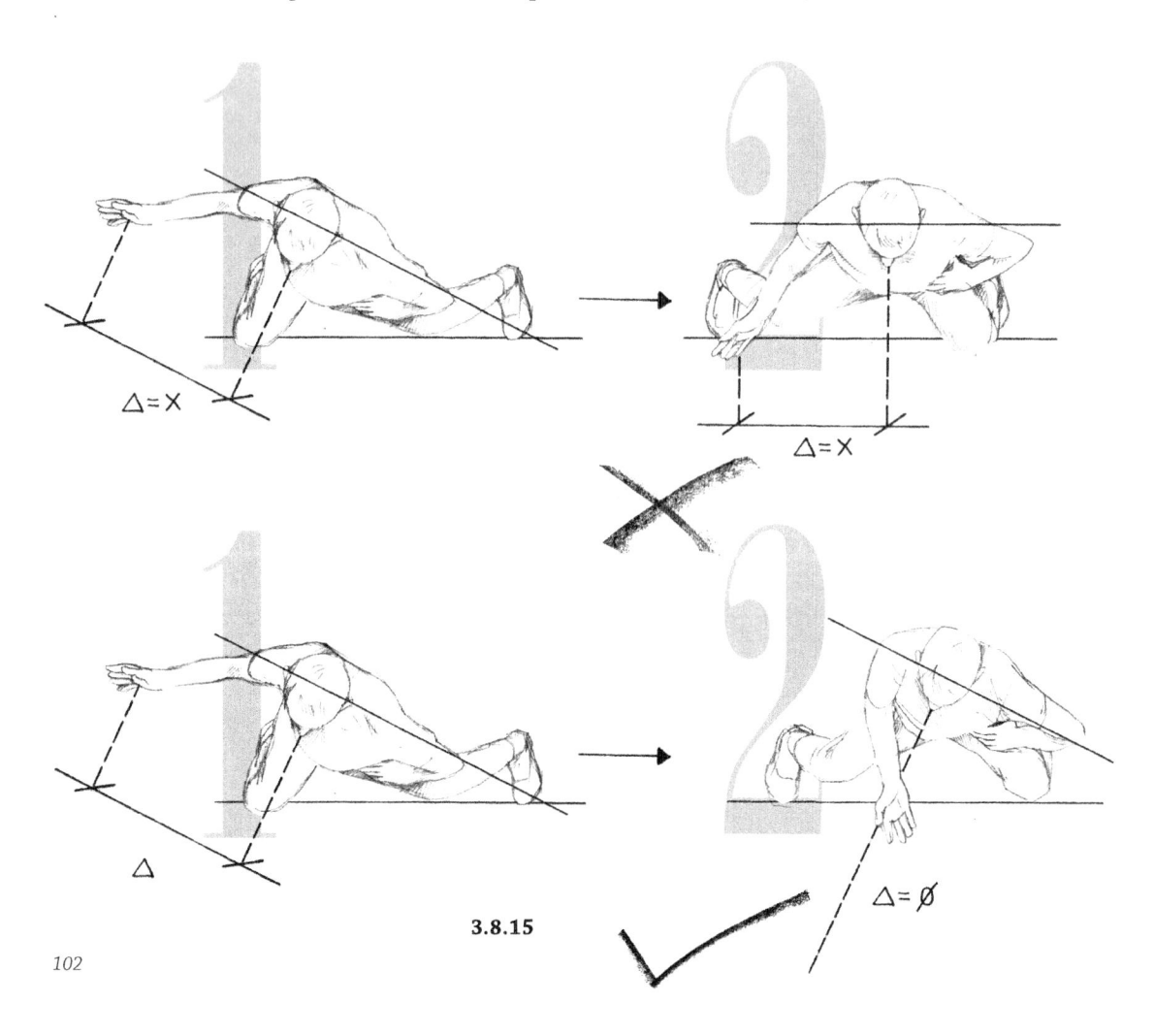

3.8.15

THE LITTLE TAIJIQUAN MANUAL FOR BEGINNERS

Only after the mechanics in the two preceding figures are well established, as shown in Figure 3.8.9, can the student progress to what 3.8.10 shows.

Here's a pretty bad mistake:

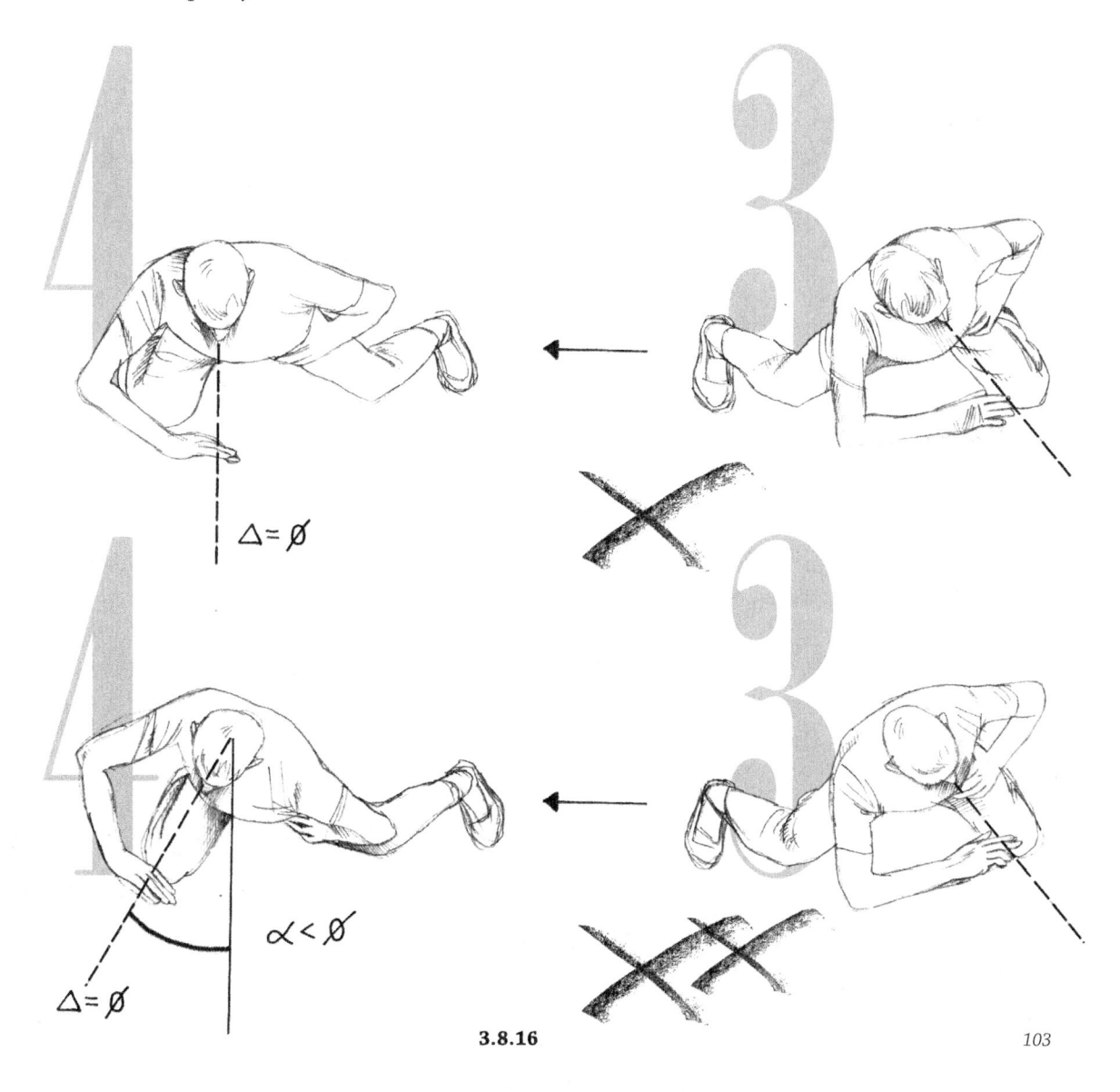

$\triangle = \emptyset$

$\triangle = \emptyset$ $\quad \alpha < \emptyset$

3.8.16

This drawing shows a beginner actively trying to turn the body, while at the same time shifting weight. In addition to not moving the hand sideways, which they should have done were the hand to follow the Dantian, the student ended up turning beyond the reference direction. In addition to not having completed the Mature Yang phase at the hand, the error shown in the upper part of the figure, the body turned into the Yin region ahead of time, as shown in the lower part of the figure.

MOVING ONWARDS

The Double Weight mistake will eventually need to be taken into account in its more refined expressions. I said that when the centre moves, hands must move following it. These words and the figures in this section can cause the beginner to move stiffly, as if the connection between the centre and the hand were too solid or hard. There is, however, a distinction between Yin and Yang between the hand and the Dantian. There should be a slight difference between them. There is a correct way to develop the perception of how this comes about, and to allow it to be a natural result of deepening practice. It is a mistake to try and force it to happen ahead of time, and it is easy to see when someone is forcing the result, if you have some experience.

A little reflection on Waisanhe will lead the reader to the conclusion that whatever is happening in the hand is also going on in the corresponding foot. If the hand is turning in one direction, the foot is turning the same way. Better said, if the upper limb is being coiled by Chansigong, the lower limb is being coiled in the same way, and just as the coiling manifests in the hand, it manifests in the foot. The foot is fixed on the ground, but internally the muscles and tendons are spiralling. The foot is stationary relative to the ground but is moving relative to the hip, as the hip is in motion. Again the same warning applies: it is a mistake to try and force it to happen. The only way to do it correctly is to relax the whole body, follow the principles, keep a good posture, and copy a good teacher.

Forms

Most people remember a predetermined sequence of movements when we mention the name Taijiquan. This is called "form". Until recently, forms were the only way to learn Taijiquan. The teaching method in the Chen family was having one's descendants repeat forms exhaustively, without much explanation, and the children would learn intuitively. When they were older and more mature, they would start receiving deeper instructions about something they were already doing naturally. If a child had a question, a relative would have the child's hands placed on their belly and demonstrate the move, and the child would directly feel how they should move.

There are several forms in Chen family Taijiquan. The main ones are:

- 9 Postures Form
- 19 Postures Form
- 38 Postures Form
- Laojia Yilu
- Laojia Erlu
- Xinjia Yilu
- Xinjia Erlu
- Broadsword
- Sword
- Spear / Staff
- Halberd
- Double Broadsword
- Double Sword

The 9, 19 and 38 Postures Forms were recently created by Chen Xiaowang due to special circumstances. They were created as the Grandmaster realized there was a need for shorter and simpler introductory forms to facilitate teaching in seminars. 38 Postures was the first one created, then 19 Postures, and very recently the 9 Postures one. This shows Chen Xiaowang's increasing efforts in making his family's art accessible and adapted to the time constraints imposed by modern life. Taijiquan teaching usually starts with the 19 Postures Form, which learning takes close to a year.

The most important form is undoubtedly Laojia Yilu, a name meaning Old Form, First Road. We refer to it as Laojia, for short. This is the form that is repeated over and over by Chen descendants, and is nicknamed Gongfu Jia, as it is the form used to build skill. The legendary Chen Fake practiced it thirty times a day, it is held as the jewel of the system. Learning the Laojia choreography usually takes about two years for non-professional students. If a student first learns the 19 Posture form, then Laojia, the time for learning Laojia drops to about a year, as 60% of movements in Laojia are included the 19 Posture form, which has become a valuable teaching tool. Laojia Erlu (Old Form, Second Road) also has nickname, Paochui or Cannon Fist. It is a fast form full of explosive movements, and therein lies its usefulness: developing speed and explosion. It is seldom seen, since performing Taijiquan's movements correctly at speed requires great skill.

The "Laojia" name for the Old First and Second Roads is relatively recent. Chen Fake, the greatest Master in Chen family's 17th generation, had moved to Beijing. He practiced many repetitions of the forms every day, and reached legendary skill levels. As his skill increased, his form gradually and spontaneously changed, and he deepened his Taijiquan. When returning to Chenjiagou, his family's village, the locals saw his forms and called them "New Forms," so the original forms started being called "Old Forms". The New Form First Road is Xinjia Yilu, and the New Form Second Road is Xinjia Erlu. They are the last forms to be learned, usually only by those having a special interest in them. Chen Fake developed Xinjia in his late fifties, when he was already a great Master, renowned for his prowess, phenomenal skill and power. Learning such a deep form before acquiring enough skill in the whole system makes no sense.

These are the free-hand forms. Taijiquan also has forms for training an apprentice in the use of traditional Chinese weapons. Those forms have great utility in body training, well beyond the use of each weapon, and a Master will know how to use each one to teach certain skills to their student, or correct their student's defects in posture and movement. The use of heavy weapons and execution at higher speed is the traditional equivalent to high intensity interval training (HIIT). Imagine practicing the Spear form in 3 or 4 minutes using a 4 or 6 kg spear, or practicing the Double Broadsword form with a 1.5 kg broadsword in each hand. It should be emphasized that before practicing with heavy weapons one must first acquire a lot of strength and skill, and close guidance from someone who knows how to do it is mandatory. Without expert guidance it is quite easy to injure oneself, and our goal, never to be forgotten, is strengthening our health.

The forms in a traditional martial arts system come from practical solutions for real situations, discovered in the course of many years, not the other way around. Primitively, there were the techniques, later on they were recorded in forms. As time went by, forms acquired more refined functions than only recording techniques, and began to occupy a more prominent place in martial arts. Repetition of Taijiquan forms is our main means of training - but not the only one.

The movements in a Taijiquan form have several functions, including technique recording. A technique (one of the "applications" of a movement) however is only efficient if you have enough strength to make it work. When the difference in strength between two opponents is too great, techniques are not that important anymore. Only when the strength of two opponents is within a range do techniques make a difference. This explains why the optimization of strength generation and transmission is so strongly emphasized in Taijiquan. Repetitive practice of forms plays a crucial role in it. Some Masters cannot hide their annoyance when a beginner student, who can barely stay a few minutes in Zhanzhuang, asks about the applications of a movement. Moreover, each movement holds many possible applications - there is not just one application per movement. A movement is actually a means of training a particular body skill. For example: when practicing Frontal Chansigong, you move one hand at a time. When practicing Two-Handed Chansigong, you move both hands at the same time, and they are always at the same height in relation to one another. When you perform the movement Hands Making Circles in Laojia, you move both hands, but they are at different heights, and when one is going up, the other one is going down. The implicit question is, how do you use your centre to command this action? Anyone can raise one arm while lowering the other, but how do you make this movement arise from the Dantian? This the skill you want to develop and perfect by practicing this movement. Any application that uses this skill, even if it looks different, can be thought of as a Hands Making Circles' application. Another example: the right hand's penultimate movement during Oblique Position corresponds to phase 4 in Chansigong, with the palm facing outwards and Qi going to the fingers. However, the weight is not shifting to the right leg as it does in Frontal Chansigong - it stays on the left leg. After much Chansigong practice, you end up wondering how it can be that the Qi goes to the right hand if the weight stays on the left leg. The answer is what you want to find when practicing the form, it is the body skill you want to develop.

For the first two years in learning, it's natural you worry about memorizing the main form, Laojia. Most people think learning Taijiquan is about memorizing the choreography composed of all those slow movements, but that is only the beginning. Actual learning only starts after the beginner memorizes the choreography, for only then questions about what is happening during the form start coming to one's mind. Soon the student realizes their path has merely begun, and that Chansigong is meant to give them a basic idea of how the body should move so Qi can circulate freely. They see Chansigong tries to show them a few movement techniques among the myriad of variations that are possible while obeying Taijiquan's principles, and a Taijiquan form is a long and continuous Silk Reeling exercise. Their job is now finding Silk Reeling within all of the form's movements. It is around this point the First Level of Gongfu ends and the Second Level begins. Only when a student can correctly use Silk Reeling in all Laojia movements are they reaching the end of the Second Level of Gongfu.

Eagerness for learning a new form is as common as for learning the so-called applications of movements. Performing martial arts moves while holding a broadsword can be very attractive. Practicing a new form with a traditional weapon can be a motivating new challenge, and promote a breakthrough in learning. One must be careful, though, not to become a forms collector, without meaningful improvement. As in everything related to Taijiquan, there is an ideal point, which is neither at one extreme nor the other, and varies according to each person. Learning new forms just because of their looks, or just for moving up in some graduation ranking, can be harmful to a specific student's technical progress. On the other hand, a Master knows how to use new forms to correct their disciple's technical problems, or to pose a new challenge that will cause their skill to leap ahead.

The speed at which a form is practiced is an interesting subject. One repetition of Laojia generally takes around 22 minutes to be completed. Like any general statement, this one won't apply in most cases: execution time varies greatly according to many factors. When one is learning a form, or has just memorized its choreography, it is natural it takes longer than usual. As one gains more familiarity, the execution time tends to decrease. When an experienced student receives important postural adjustments, they will intuitively try to transpose these adjustments into the form. This creates a need for the form to be "relearned", that is, even though the choreography remains the same, the body mechanics for performing the movements has changed. This is poetically referred to as "always the same spring, always different flowers". When such a change occurs, the execution time usually increases. Then it gradually drops until it reaches the usual time for that student. Conversely, it can also happen that with a change in the body mechanics the movements become better linked, and the execution time falls. I have seen Masters practicing one round of Laojia as fast as in 12 minutes, and as slow as in 45 minutes. Practicing one round of Laojia in 45 minutes while keeping the movements fluid and continuous is quite difficult. It also strengthens the legs a lot, and is more appropriate for meditative practices. Practicing one round in 12 minutes is nearly four times faster, which means that in the same practice time, one trains four times the number of punches, four times the number of kicks, four times the number of each technique. Legend has it that Chen Fake could do one Laojia in six minutes.

After a few years of practice, we can finally talk about Chansigong as it should be. The preceding drawings and explanations are helpful up to a point, but we need to understand that the resolution employed is too coarse to convey what should actually happen. Once again imagine we are trying to describe day and night from the viewpoint of Yin-Yang. I could say: day is Yang, night is Yin. Soon this would be taken as too limited a description, and I would have to speak of the Four Appearances and their correspondence with times of noon, six o'clock, midnight, and six o'clock in the morning. Instead of one bit, I now have two bits of information as a representation of my universe: this would be a higher resolution description. I could then indefinitely increase my observation's resolution, and describe the proportion of Yin and Yang at every instant of a day. I would need a large volume of information to precisely define each instant. Here's an example:

3.9.1

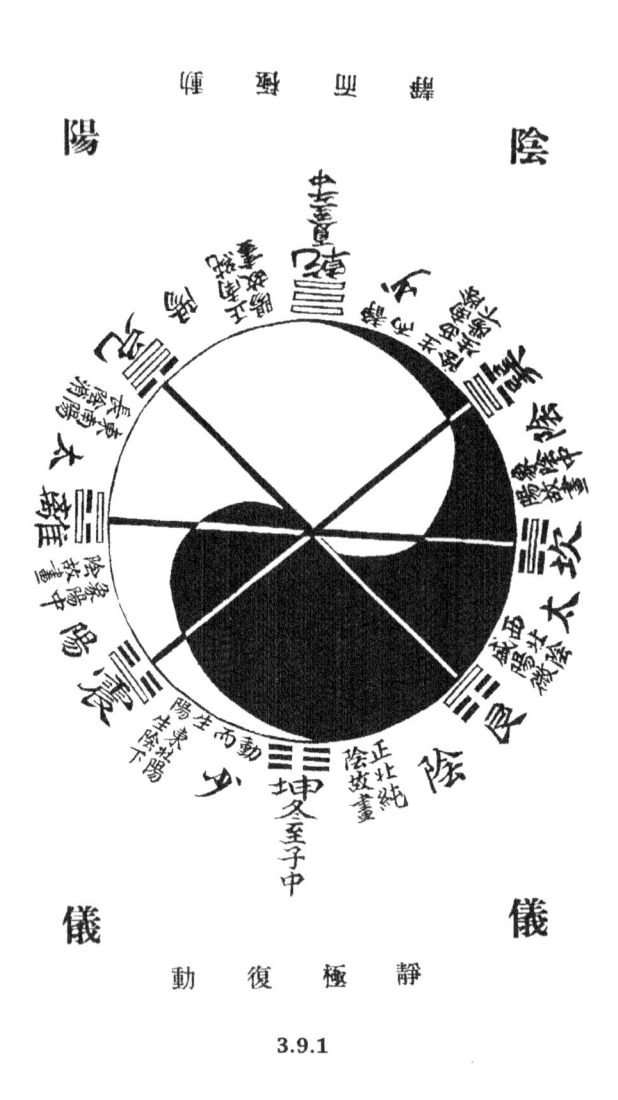

I'm using 3 bits of information, or in the symbology chosen by the Yi Jing, three lines. With 3 bits I can pinpoint 8 instants in time or 8 instants in the waxing and waning of Yin and Yang. In the following drawings, you can see 8 instants in Double Hand Chansigong:

THE LITTLE TAIJIQUAN MANUAL FOR BEGINNERS

3.9.2   **1**   **2**

3.9.3   **3**   **4**

111

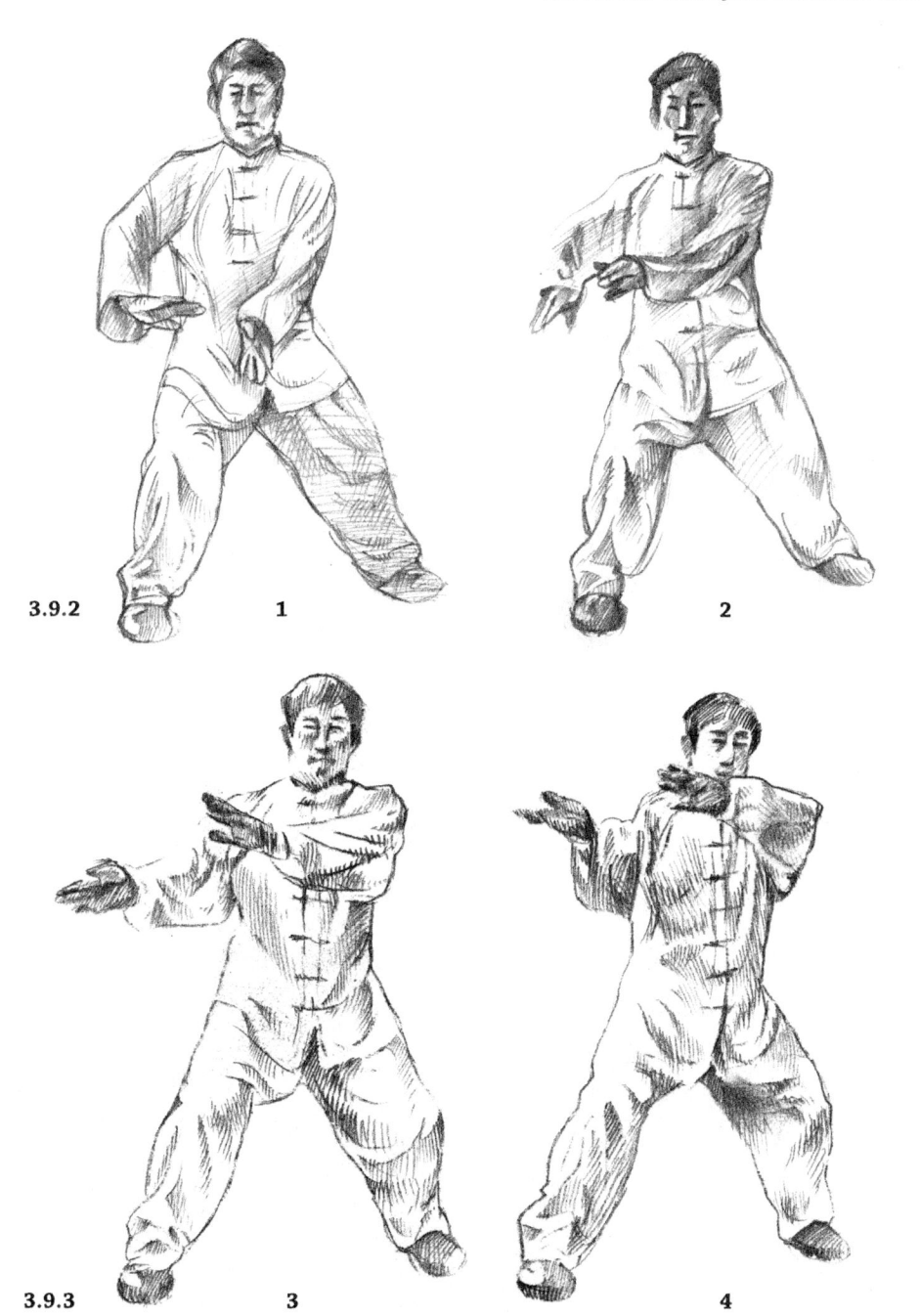

THE LITTLE TAIJIQUAN MANUAL FOR BEGINNERS

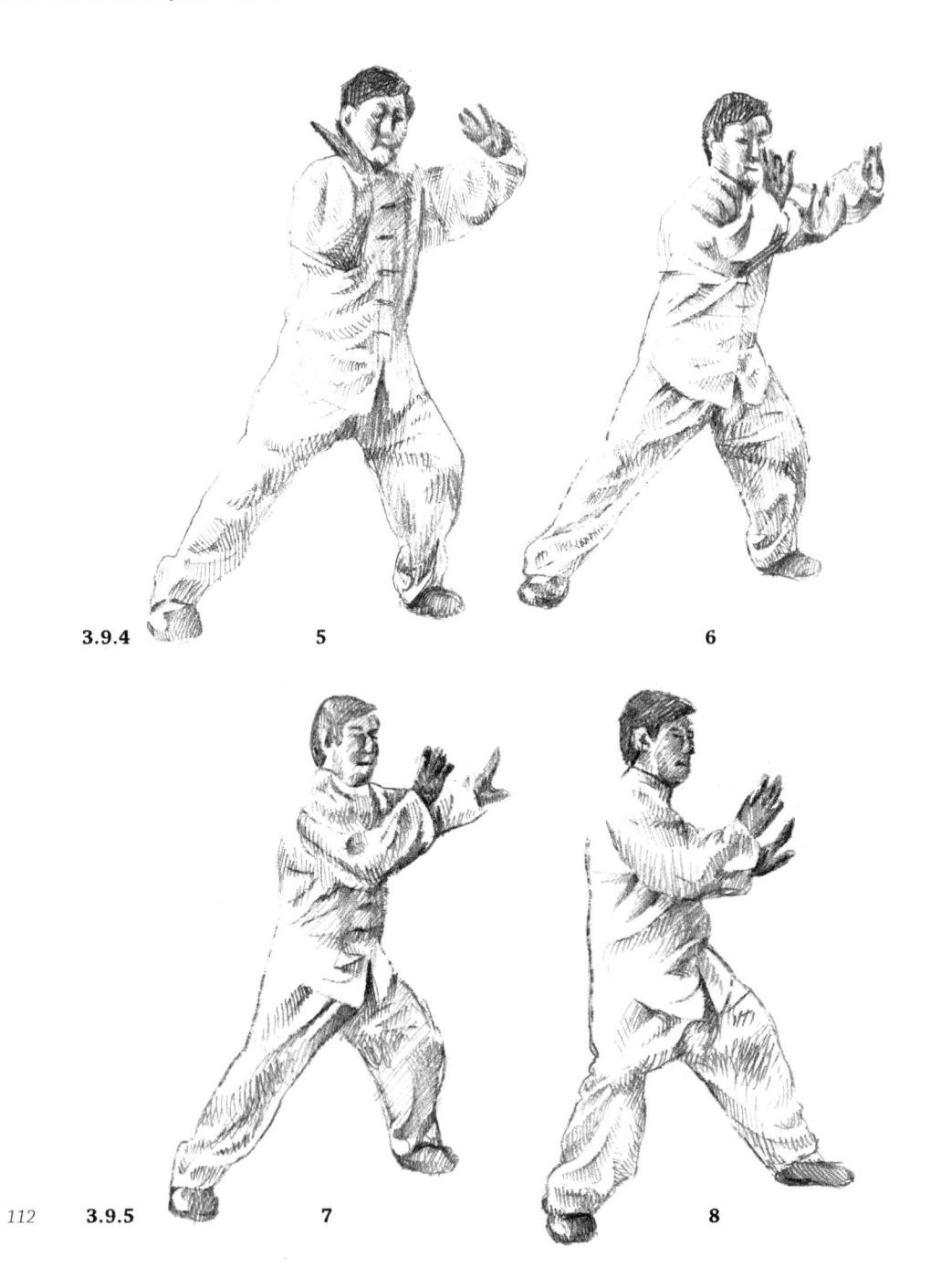

3.9.4   5   6

3.9.5   7   8

You may have noticed that using 3 bits of information corresponds to the Eight Trigrams in the Yi Jing. The Classic of Changes shows hexagrams, that is, 6 bit information sets, or six lines, to describe the changing from Yin to Yang and vice versa. In the Yi Jing's text it is explained each line can be "fixed" or "mobile", meaning each is stable or unstable, they can change in the next instant or not. The Yi Jing thus details 4,096 possible configurations between maximum Yin and maximum Yang. A figure with only 128 configurations is shown next:

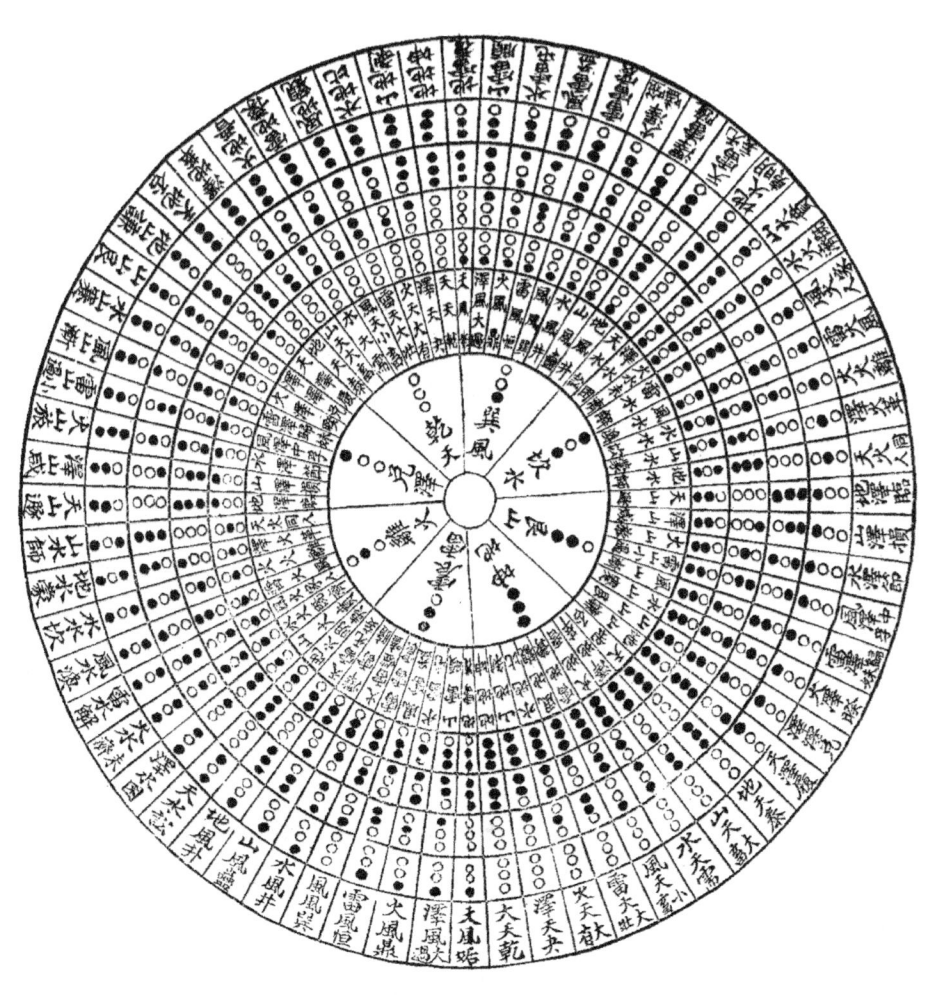

3.9.6

Sounds like it is too complex, but it is much closer to our daily life than we first assume. Think of Meteorology: we never hesitate to state there are four seasons in the year, and to correlate them to the Four Appearances. It is a trivial example. It is in fact a huge simplification of our everyday reality. The way temperature and rainfall vary is not linear at all, there are several overlapping cycles, and many variables such as local microclimate interfere continuously. We nevertheless talk about spring, summer, autumn and winter as an acceptable generalization and as a didactic resource even in low latitudes where seasons are not well defined. Chansigong fulfills precisely this role in regard to forms. Another way of looking at this issue is saying learning Taijiquan is like learning calligraphy. We think vaguely about this, we remember the famous complementarity between "Pen and Sword", and leave it there. The link is much closer: how many years does it take a child to learn how to write? Someone might hastily answer "one or two," but an expert would say it takes something like 7 or 8 years, because they will count the years it took the child to acquire the motor coordination necessary for the task, not just the years of formal training in writing at school. A good way to reflect on learning Taijiquan is by observing children between zero and eight years old - I suggest you really try to find an opportunity to do it. Take a few minutes to observe a newborn, and you will see that they have virtually no motor control. They can't even close one hand independently, when they close one, often both hands close. They very slowly gain motor coordination on a daily basis, gradually achieving great feats along the way: standing and walking. One day they manage to hold a spoon, but aiming well at the mouth is a difficult task, and half the food misses the target. Years go by, and by the time a child reaches first grade, they have enough control to hold a pencil, but they still can't colour a shape inside its lines. By the time they leave second grade, they can draw letters in cursive writing and plan the size of letters in relation to the space provided. When their journey began, their hands knew only two states: either fully contracted, holding something tightly, or almost completely lax. Completely Yang, or completely Yin. Over time, they learned to use their hands within a continuum, in a less quantized fashion, until the control became spontaneous and they no longer think about it when writing. The same motor training happens when you learn Taijiquan. At first, during Chansigong, your hands are either too taut or too flaccid. When the teacher asks you to relax a little, your hands become too soft. In time, they become able to keep some structure while simultaneously relaxing. This doesn't happen exclusively to the hands, as when writing - it happens to the whole body, especially to the body's centre. When practicing, you are actively seeking to develop in your body's centre the same motor progress a child experiences in their hands when learning to write.

The understanding of how Yin and Yang express in the body evolves with deepening practice. In the beginning, it was enough to know that the upper body is Yang, and the lower body is Yin; that the back is Yang, and the front is Yin. With time one realizes the head is more Yang than the chest, the chest is more Yang than the abdomen. The feet are more Yin than the thighs, which are more Yin than the abdomen. Similarly, the energy channels mapped by Acupuncture are not simply Yin or Yang, they are organized into six energetic levels, namely, from the most Yang to the most Yin: Tai Yang, Shao Yang, Yang Ming, Tai Yin, Jue Yin, Shao Yin. We have just described Yin and Yang in your body, using one direction at a time (first vertical, then horizontal), but the two directions are present at the same time in the body. This creates two opposite spirals, which manifest on the ventral and dorsal faces in a complementary fashion, as one would expect:

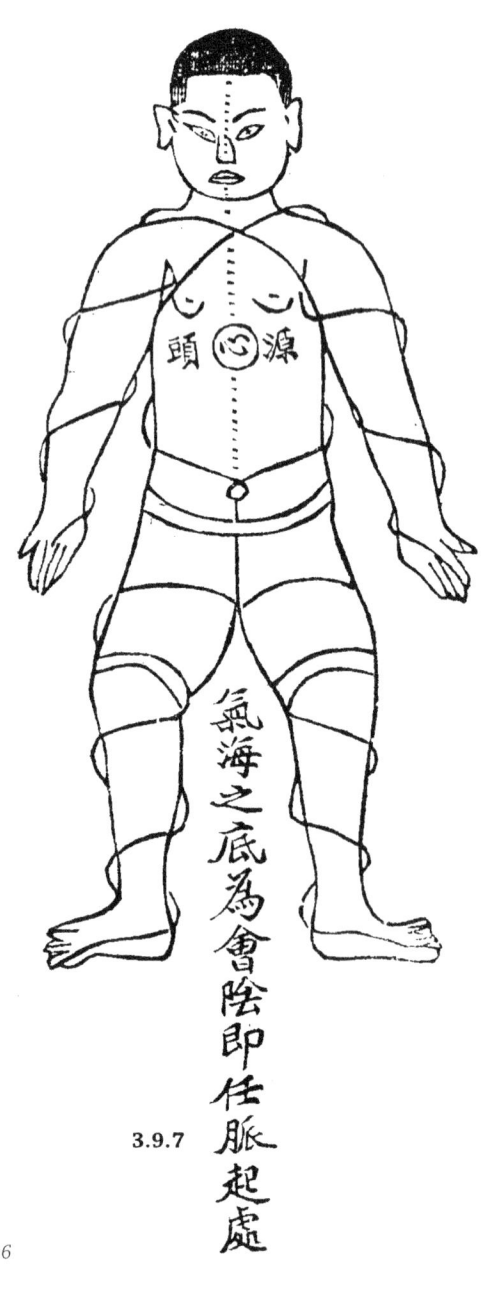

THE LITTLE TAIJIQUAN MANUAL FOR BEGINNERS

氣海之底為會陰即任脈起處

3.9.7

督脈通前蛋絃為海底

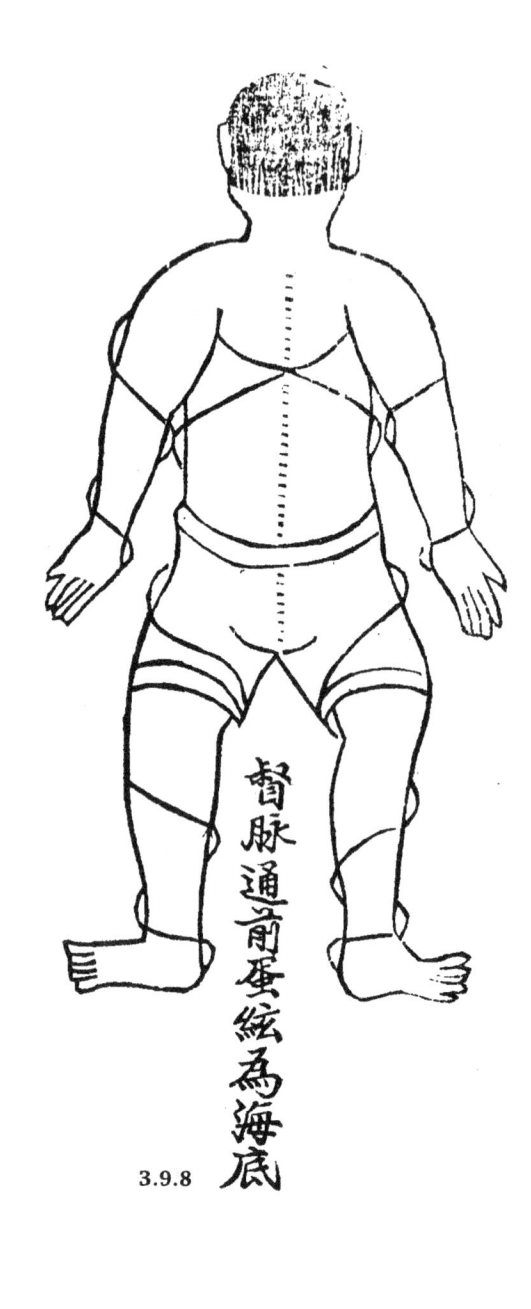

3.9.8

This is an analysis of the static body. The spirals are always present, even during movement, because they are part of the body's physical structure. The Chansigong Qi circulation is superimposed on this background.

All of this is way too complex to be voluntarily implemented in movement practice. The only chance of learning how to move the body using all this information is by relaxing the body, keeping the posture taught during Zhanzhuang, and following someone who knows how to do it. This is why it is so important to follow a Master when practicing. Your brain and body are able to copy a Master's movements better than you can imagine, because they do it intuitively, without the rational mind's direct interference. When a student with enough previous training follows a high level Master, they usually feel "something magical", and get a very motivating feeling of having improved a lot in a few minutes. When the Master stops demonstrating and asks the student to practice by themselves, the feeling lasts for a few minutes, and then disappears. Your body can copy that magical something while the Master is showing it, but it is not skilled enough to keep it. Practicing and trying to remember the feeling to get their body to improve in the direction shown by the Master is up to the student.

This brings us to a reflection on the current teaching model. When a seminar teaching model is adopted, questions arise for beginners and advanced students alike: the former wonder why attend a seminar where they will be taught a long form that they may not be able to memorize, the latter wonder why attend a seminar where they will be taught a form they already know. The answer is the same: the goal of training is not learning the form. The goal of Taijiquan training is changing the body so it naturally moves in a new way.

It's only possible to transform your body and change the way it moves through direct contact with a Master. Forms are important, but they are not Taijiquan itself, they are the means by which Taijiquan is taught. If you do not know the form that will be taught in a seminar, and it seems long and complex, this should not be a reason for discouragement. Concentrate on trying to remember the feeling in your body after you are adjusted by the Master, and try to copy not only the choreography, but the way the Master moves - for this is the main teaching. If you already know the form to be taught, this is a great reason to attend a seminar, as you can direct all your attention to the posture adjustments you will receive and to how to move the body.

The best way to learn Taijiquan is through daily and prolonged master-disciple contact. However, moving to China's countryside for several years is not an option for most people. The solution is attending annual seminars with Chen family Masters. On the other hand, learning only in seminars is often not enough, you also need to take regular classes with a teacher with a more advanced skill level than you.

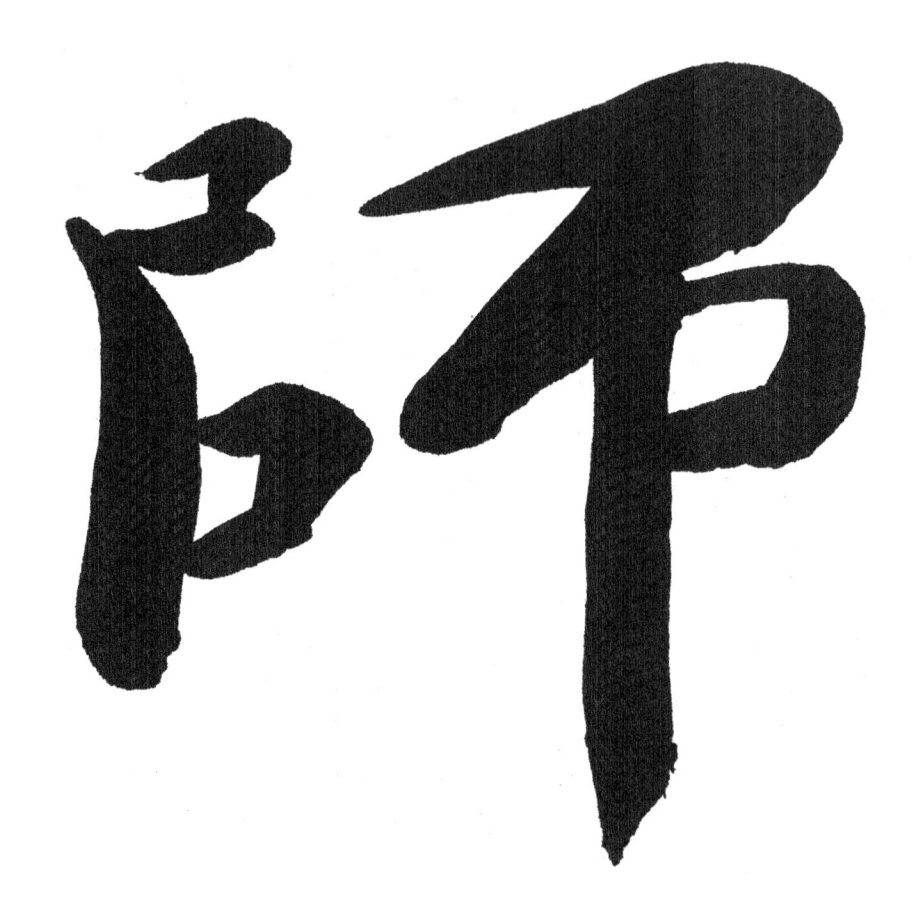

Shīfù (師父): shī 師, teacher, instructor, combined to fù 父, father: in modern Chinese, Master, the transmitter of secret knowledges. Contrast to lǎoshī 老師, "old (a word conveying respect) teacher", honourable teacher, the term for referring to teachers of publicly available knowledge.

父

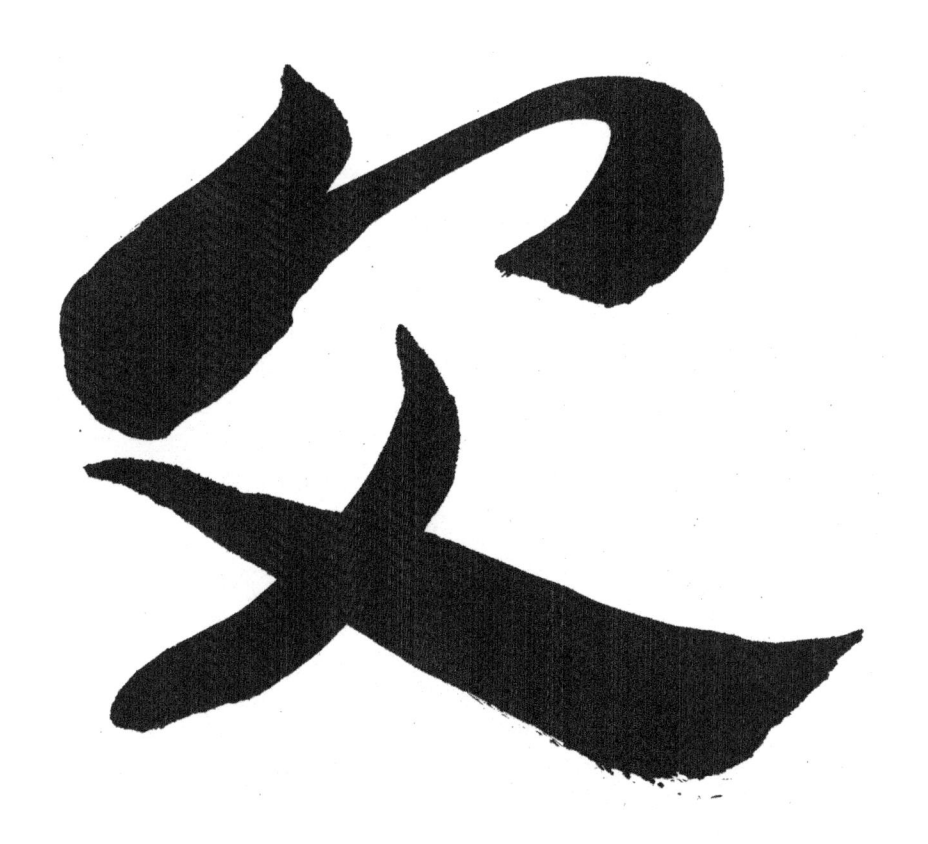

Masters' Teachings

Listen carefully

Listen attentively to every word I say. Every word coming out my mouth is the result of 20 years of exhaustive practice, day and night training and reflecting about Taijiquan.
— Chen Yingjun

Chen Yingjun told me this once, when I took too long to follow a technical instruction of his. As the years pass and hours of practice accumulate, I understand better each of his instructions, and his way of teaching his art. It becomes ever clearer how broad his sight is, and how carefully considered each instruction is in its content and precise timing, so to produce the best didactic effect on the student. An example: he did not want me to practice one of the forms in the system for many years. I willingly obeyed, because I have total confidence in him, his technical skill and his purity of purpose. Today I can see exactly why he chose this path for me, and I clearly feel that following his guidance was much more productive for my progress than any other alternative.

Living teachings

The teaching is alive.
— Chen Yingjun

After his 2013 seminar in Rio de Janeiro, I asked Master Chen Yingjun why he had taught a Taijiquan topic in a different way than I was used to seeing him do. The technical content was the same, but his didactic had changed. This was his answer, and he explained further:

Students change, I change, and conditions change.
— Chen Yingjun

We'd expect the students to change, because that's what they are practicing for. We usually don't think about how much a Master changes with the years, however, as the "Master" title conveys a sense of accomplishment — but a Taijiquan Master is also practicing intensively, and since their skill level is very high, they improve quicker than we could imagine. Seeing improvement in a Master is difficult for a beginner, first because it takes place on a very subtle level, invisible to the student; secondly because the student thinks on too small a time scale. If you compare Chen Xiaowang's videos from the 1980s to a recent one, the difference is striking.

Any given Taijiquan seminar can have very different conditions compared to another one: number of students, their average level, the heterogeneity of the group, which form is being taught. All this requires adaptation from the teacher, the better they are, the better they will be able to change their didactics to benefit their students.

It's easier to teach a child

It is easier to teach a child because their mind is like a blank canvas.
— Chen Yingjun

When adults start learning Taijiquan, they already have a collection of preconceived ideas about what it is, maybe even about some of its technical aspects. This is all the more true, if they have read about it before, or practiced another martial arts style. Almost any idea brought to class tends to make learning more difficult. The one exception may be experience in meditation. Taijiquan is a very un-obvious art, with innumerable depth levels, and a very unique approach to body mechanics.

When children start learning, even if they have some previous experience, they are naturally more open to learning. If a child is four or five years old, they will learn with a completely pure heart, and their mind will be free to take in information. This is the attitude we should adopt when learning Taijiquan: complete non-attachment to what we think we already know.

There's a very concrete reason for this. Say you are learning the posture "Hand Hides Arm and Fist". The first reaction most people have is thinking, "oh, that's a punch". If that thought sticks, you will not only miss the other applications of this move, but your body will try to throw a punch in the way you already know. If, on the other hand, you had never seen a punch before, and had no idea what a punch is, you'd do your best to simply copy the way the teacher moves – which is precisely what you should do anyway.

Do only one thing

In a seminar in Brazil, one of my students, upon seeing Master Chen Yingjun demonstrate Laojia for the first time, was astonished by his skill. He asked the Master during question time how one could achieve such a deep Gongfu. Chen Yingjun replied:

You must do only one thing.
— *Chen Yingjun*

He meant that the student should devote himself to only one art, whatever it was, if he wished to reach a high level.

Naturalness

Naturalness is the first principle.
— *Chen Xiaowang*

The Huangdi Neijing Suwen is the oldest classic text in Chinese Medicine, believed to have been written around five centuries before Christ. It is organized in the form of Emperor Huangdi's questions to his court physician, Qi Bo. Asked why men were no longer healthy and died prematurely, Qi Bo replied (according to Paul Unschuld's translation, 1-2-1):

The people of high antiquity,
those who knew the Way,
they modelled [their behaviour] on yin and yang and they complied with the arts
and the calculations.

Unschuld translated Dao as "Way". What does it mean to know the Dao? In the Daodejing ch. 25 we read:

ren fa di di fa tian tian fa dao dao fa zi ran

Man follows earth, earth follows heaven, heaven follows Dao, and Dao follows itself - sometimes translated as "the method of the Dao is naturalness."

In other words, the teaching of Grandmaster Chen Xiaowang is in perfect harmony with the Neijing's statement. But what does naturalness mean? It is certainly not doing whatever suits each one. Naturalness means following the laws of nature, the method of Dao.

One Yin, one Yang, this is Dao

Dao unfolds in the manifest world into Yin and Yang. Naturalness thus means conforming to the laws governing interaction of Yin and Yang. If carefully observing nature, one sees day and night, winter and summer, inspiration and expiration are direct expressions of it.

Chen Xiaowang's teaching therefore does not mean Taijiquan should be practiced to cater to each student's individual wishes - there is no such thing resembling "to practice Taijiquan my own way". The technical principles are always there, precisely defined, guiding one's practice.

In one of the Grandmaster's seminars in Brazil, a student asked him why practicing so much was necessary, if naturalness is Taijiquan's first principle. He answered:

If it were only natural, there would be no need to practice.
First practice, then it becomes natural.
— *Chen Xiaowang*

Taijiquan fully respects the human body's natural, physiological movement. No antiphysiological twisting or stretching is done during practice, as these would make the relaxation needed for good practice impossible. Breathing should remain natural, and should never be forced, for it will spontaneously conform to the needs and possibilities of the student. Adjustment of breath to movement is a natural process, which takes a long time and occurs very gradually. The mind should be partly free, partly concentrated: practice itself and the attention needed for refining movement will lead to a natural state of mindfulness. Finally, the whole body's inner strength can only be developed naturally, one cannot force its development. All that can be done is keeping correct posture and relaxing the whole body, allowing the natural emergence of strength. In Zhanzhuang practice, for example, the teacher adjusts the student's body's posture, then the student keeps the posture. There is nothing the student can or should do except stand still, since the teacher has adjusted the posture to make the student's joints as free as possible. In order for the student to keep the posture the body has to exert force against gravity. This force however should not be consciously induced or commanded by the student, it should be natural and spontaneous. If the student were to try and command this force, they would exert it the way they are accustomed to, not the way the teacher wants them to learn.

The teacher follows the student

First, the teacher follows the student. Then, the student follows the teacher.
— *Chen Xiaowang*

When beginning to teach, a teacher must know that the student will not follow their instructions - not because they don't want to, but because their body cannot do it. If it were possible for the student to absorb and reproduce the teaching as soon as it is offered, they would no longer need a teacher after the first lesson. Taijiquan Masters are so patient because they understand the extent of transformation necessary in the student's body for them to move correctly.

You can't teach a skill

It is impossible to teach the skill. You can only show the way.
— *Chen Yingjun*

    Chen Yingjun taught me this during a conversation about how to teach Taijiquan. Common sense would be that one goes to a class to receive knowledge. This view might stem from our consumerism culture - it would be as if one could buy knowledge. Advertisements usually emphasize the (false) appearance that going to class and paying tuition would be enough for "graduating".

    This is not how it works in a traditional art. Knowledge is transmitted within a master-disciple relationship (here we're not referring to the instructor's skill level, instead to the mode of transmission). One doesn't go to a Taijiquan class to receive knowledge, but to learn how to practice. It is the way of cultivating knowledge that is taught. A teacher can only point the direction, and help correct deviations. It is through dedicated practice that genuine knowledge in the art can be attained. That is the essence of Gongfu.

Relaxation and posture

First, keep your posture. Secondly, relax.
— Chen Yingjun

This instruction was given in Magdeburg, in 2016, when Chen Yingjun was explaining what relaxing means in Taijiquan. The point is that relaxing too much is possible and in fact quite easy. He was telling students they should keep the posture he would put them in during Zhanzhuang first of all - and then, without losing their postural adjustment, they should relax. When a Master adjusts your posture in Zhanzhuang or in one of the form's postures, your body develops power according to Taijiquan's principles, respecting Waisanhe. If you lose the postural adjustment, even by a few millimetres, you will lose the optimal alignment, and will not know how to find it again. Therefore, when you try to relax in a posture, you should care not to overdo it.

The cause of strengthening

You become strong because of relaxation, not in spite of it.
— *Chen Yingjun*

Chen Yingjun told me this when he once noticed I was hesitant to relax. It is common to find the repeated instructions to relax strange, up to a certain point in learning, because when relaxing we may feel we are developing less power. This is also true only up to a certain point in learning. After a while, our body learns strength and relaxation do not exclude each other, they are expressions of Yin and Yang, so they generate each other.

Breathing

If you have wrong posture and wrong breathing, you have only one mistake; if you have wrong posture and correct breathing, you have two mistakes.
— Chen Xiaowang

This teaching means that breathing should be according to your posture. If your posture is wrong - as it is in anyone who is not a Master - your breathing should be wrong in the same way as your posture is, so that they be in harmony with each other. There will then be only one mistake. If your posture is wrong, but your breath is "correct" with respect to some standard, your breath will not be in harmony with your posture. There will then be two errors: the postural error, and the error of discordance between breath and posture. What is the best way to adjust your breathing? You should let your breathing become completely natural. Your body knows what to do much better than you do in this respect. Just keep gradually improving your posture with practice, and your breathing will improve the same.

With Qi only

If you were to only use Qi, you wouldn't even get out of bed in the morning.
— *Chen Xiaowang*

There is a huge mystification around Qi in the West. Chen Xiaowang explains that Qi alone is actually very weak. You can't perform concrete actions with Qi alone. Qi is used in Taijiquan to direct the body's power. A Master uses his energy circulation as kind of a guide, so their movement and posture generate the maximum possible physical strength.

Best time for practice

The best time of the day for practicing Taijiquan is from eleven o'clock in the evening until one o'clock in the morning.
— *Chen Yingjun*

Some believe Taijiquan must be practiced early in the morning and late in the afternoon, since it's common to see people practicing in parks during those hours. This is simply the most convenient time: it doesn't coincide with most people's working hours, and it avoids the sun on students' heads. In winter, you may find students practicing outdoors between 10am and 4pm in countries with a cold climate, as these are the warmest hours.

The best time of day to practice is from eleven o'clock in the evening until one o'clock in the morning because this is the time when Yin is strongest in nature, and when a person's mind is quietest and calms down most easily. In many meditation systems this time is described as "the hour of return", and symbolizes the attainment of the greatest concentration. By practicing at this time one takes advantage of the natural order to which man is inevitably bound. The only problem is, this is also the best time to be asleep!

It is necessary to change

One of the first times I met Chen Xiaowang, I had a question about Fengshui for which I couldn't find an answer. Some systems for choosing Acupuncture points are based on cardinal directions and their relationship to the seasons and stars. China is in the Northern Hemisphere, and there was no literature at the time recommending or not changes for the Southern Hemisphere, where I lived then. I asked the Grandmaster about it, and he replied:

A teacher teaches pronouns to the student at school:
"I am the teacher, you are the student, he is your father."
The student goes home and says to the father, "I am the teacher, you are the student, he is your father," when he should say, "He is the teacher, I am the student, you are the father."
Change is necessary.
— *Chen Xiaowang*

Leave your neck out of it

The weight should sink as if you were hanging by a thread at the top of your head - but leave your neck out of it.
— *Chen Yingjun*

When asked by a student about the traditional instruction saying "sink as if hanging by a thread," Chen Yingjun replied thusly - because the student who asked the question stretched his neck upwards. The traditional instruction is correct, but one must know how to interpret it. One should not stretch the neck, as this will cause tension throughout the whole body. There is an ideal position for the cervical spine in each person, but a Master has to adjust your body and your cranium's position so you are able to feel it.

Do not pull your knees out

If you pull your knees out, they will not engage properly, and your legs will not be used.
— *Chen Yingjun*

    A fellow practitioner saw me talking to Chen Yingjun about knee alignment , and joined our talk, contributing a question about why many people seem to pull their knees out. Pulling the knees outwards is a widespread mistake. If one does it, part of the load that should be borne by the musculature is shifted to the joint's tendons. Not only is the leg not used as it should, but one can create problems in the knee.

Feet position

When asked whether the toes should be open or forward during Zhanzhuang, Grandmaster Chen Xiaowang replied:

If you walk like this [showing open toes], practice like this. If you walk like this [showing toes pointing forward], practice like this.
— Chen Xiaowang

Forcing your toes to point forward or your feet to be parallel is counterproductive. First of all, feet position is mainly dependent on the hip joints. If you force your feet to an arbitrary position, you may cause joint pain, and you will certainly create unnecessary tension. Your feet position will change naturally as your posture improves.

Teacher's skill

Either you have skill, or you don't.
— *Chen Yingjun*

    I once asked my Shifu if he could show me how to teach a student something. This was his answer. He meant you can't teach something you haven't understood. How much a teacher can impart is necessarily limited by their skill level.

Focus

50% concentrated, 50% not.
50% of the mind on the Dantian, 50% on the whole body.
— *Chen Xiaowang*

Two of the most common questions when Chen Xiaowang was teaching in Brazil were: should I concentrate or not, after all? Where should I focus my mind? Taijiquan offers you a meditation method that's a little different than one might think. Our expectations when we hear about meditation is that we must force the mind to focus. Such methods exist, they may also be good, but this is not the way in Taijiquan, which first principle is naturalness. In order to progress towards a meditative state in Taijiquan, we change the body so it provides the conditions for meditation to be naturally achieved. On the other hand, you should not let your mind simply wander around while you practice. A little direction is needed. Chen Xiaowang says, half concentrated, half free. Just as there is a middle path between muscle tension and laxity, there is a middle path between forcing your mind and letting it wander. The art lies in finding this path.

Trying to copy what you can't do

If you try to copy something you cannot do, you will be doing it wrong.
— Chen Yingjun

Learning Taijiquan largely involves copying your teacher. There are, however, some things one should try to copy, and other things one should not try. A good example is a student seeing a Master demonstrating a low posture in a photograph, and trying to copy his posture exactly, particularly when the Master's thighs look a little rotated outwards. Chen Yingjun explains that in order to be able to do this, a practitioner must already have reached a very high level, and when a Master takes such a picture, they have been training for decades. Many changes have already taken place in their legs after so much training. Trying to copy something like that is a mistake and will cause problems.

Posture height

It's not how low you get in a posture - it's how well aligned you are. First do it right. Then do it low.
— *Chen Yingjun*

    Chen Yingjun is often asked why he usually raises his students' posture in seminars when adjusting them in Zhanzhuang. He explains anyone can just push you down in a posture, but he, on the other hand, is trying to teach something special: how to align the body correctly. Therefore, the height of a posture is secondary - it's often better for learning to have the student reduce the physical load so they can get better alignment.

First, Qi returns to Dantian

When Qi can return from the whole body to the Dantian, Qi can flow from the Dantian to the whole body. This is pengjin.
— *Chen Xiaowang*

This sentence from Grandmaster Chen Xiaowang is a profound description of Taijiquan's way of generating power. Pengjin is often translated as "repelling power", however this is only one possible translation, and reveals only a restricted meaning. Pengjin, in a broader sense as explained by the Grandmaster, refers to the way the body is structured and generates relaxed power, and to how Qi circulates freely complementing this. It is crucial to note that the teaching starts by talking about the return of Qi to the Dantian. Qi can only return if the body is trained to relax. Only if Qi can return, can it flow from the centre to the entire body. Here it is important to stress Qi circulation is a natural feature of the human body, there is no need to force it - correct alignment and movement are sufficient. Training the body to move in a natural and relaxed way, eliminating blockages for Qi's return, is all that is needed for it to flow naturally.

Relaxing a muscle that is tense begets two effects: it is unlocked, and the antagonist muscle naturally starts working. These two effects allow the involved joints to return to their physiological positions, in turn allowing free flow of Qi.

Contrary to what a beginner assumes, one does not train in sending Qi to the hand. One trains in allowing unimpeded return of Qi (through relaxation). The flow of Qi to the palm (or any other part) happens naturally with correct posture and correct movement.

Don't look for feelings

Don't seek for Qi feelings when practicing, this is a mistake. Look for the right way to practice, and Qi will increase naturally. The more you look for Qi, the less you will feel it.
— Chen Yingjun

A frequent question afflicting those who start to practice Taijiquan is what Qi circulation feels like. Qi feeling is usually described as a warm flow through the trunk and limbs, according to the movement. For example, in Frontal Chansigong, warmth would follow the path: body's centre - up the back - shoulder - arm - elbow - hand - arm - hip - body's centre. This description can cause many misunderstandings. You should know that when you start practicing it is quite common to feel something like it, but after a few months of practice the feelings usually disappear. This is because the initial sensation is simply due to an improvement in peripheral blood circulation, nothing more. When the body gets used to it, the new feeling goes away.

Chen Yingjun explains one must not practice in order to obtain a feeling, because feelings are not the goal. The goal in Taijiquan practice is the development of integral strength, of Gongfu, and strengthening health as consequence. Appearance and disappearance of physical sensations during the path towards these goals are temporary side effects without much relevance.

We can further clarify using a Chinese Medicine parallel: when receiving Acupuncture, a patient may have various feelings at the point where a needle is inserted (tingling, itching, heaviness) or in the energy channel. These feelings are generally referred to as "arrival of Qi". The goal of a consultation is not obtaining these sensations, but the restoration of balance and consequently of health. If a patient has many sensations but their health state remains the same, nothing has been achieved by the Acupuncturist. Likewise in Taijiquan: the student can feel many different things, but if they can't show concrete results, nothing will have been achieved.

One should also not look for sensations when practicing, for a very simple reason: sensations are expected to change as the student's skill improves. How could someone practicing for five years have the same feelings as someone practicing for a year? If this were to happen, it would mean the person practicing for longer is still at the same level as the person practicing for less time. Someone seeking a sensation will be stuck, it will become a hindrance to their progress. Sensations often change during the first few years of practice.

One should seek to follow Taijiquan's principles instead, keep a good posture, and acquire relaxation and stability.

Pain

Where there is pain, there is blockage. Where there is no blockage, there is no pain.
— *Chen Xiaowang*

This teaching is one of the principles in Chinese Medicine rationale: pain is caused by the blockage of Qi circulation. On the other hand, where there is no blockage, there is no pain. An interesting example is the treatment of a herniated intervertebral disc through Acupuncture. In many cases, Acupuncture is able to eliminate pain and numbness caused by a herniated disc, and the Medical Doctor overseeing the case may choose to withdraw a recommendation for surgery. Acupuncture does not "heal" the herniation proper, as the intervertebral disc's protrusion is not reversed. Acupuncture restores Qi's circulation, causing the decreasing or disappearance of symptoms.

Similarly in Taijiquan, pain is a symptom of Qi's circulation blockage. Whenever Qi's passage is impeded, there will be pain - whenever the student feels pain they must know Qi's passage is impeded in that area. It is important however to underline that perception of pain is often confused with muscle tiredness or the burning exercise causes - the Grandmaster does not mean tiredness or burning, he means sharp or acute pain. It's natural the muscles get very tired during Taijiquan. In a private class with the Grandmaster it's common to feel the muscles in whole body are exhausted, but there's no pain. This feeling is somewhat surprising the first times it occurs, because in ordinary exercises, when fatigue arrives pain usually accompanies it, since the posture is not perfect in terms of Qi circulation. Not in Taijiquan. In good quality Taijiquan all musculature is proportionally used and the whole body is exercised, at the same time there are no Qi circulation blockages.

Raise your average

You practice to raise your average.
— Chen Yingjun

  I once asked Chen Yingjun about the natural ups and downs in skill and power during the course of time. There are days when we move better, and there are days when we feel very stiff and can't seem to move at all. How could someone be always ready to use their Taijiquan? This was his answer.

Light arms

When the arms are light, it is as if there were no arms. Then you can turn.
— Chen Yingjun

The most fundamental instructions in Taijiquan are given at the start of Zhanzhuang practice. They are: keep the body straight, relax the whole body.

An incorrect understanding of the second instruction's meaning may lead the student to move the arms heavily. On the other hand, the student's desire to strengthen the body may induce them to try to perform movements with brute force, or exertion, during the explosive movements. Both are serious mistakes which prevent the body from freely turning.

Commonly spread incorrect perceptions are: there must be weight on the arms when performing the movements, relaxation leads to the feeling of weight, and that during Tuishou the relaxed arms should weigh on the opponent. All these perceptions are wrong and prevent correct movement, because they are expressions of double weight.

The student should feel their arms during Taijiquan movements as if they were weightless. The arms will be supported by the trunk, and not suspended from the shoulder muscles: this is the way to relax arms, without holding weight on top of the body. Weight should always be on the student's feet as a result of correct posture. There should be no blockages or deviations loading any joints. Qi and Jin should reach the arms and hands, not weight.

Speed of practice

If you practice too slowly, Qi stops.
— *Chen Yingjun*

Chen Yingjun told me that when he once saw me practicing too slowly in his backyard. Chen Family Taijiquan's forms and Chansigong can be practiced at various speeds. There is no ready-made formula. The above quoted "too slow" meant too slow for me, at that time. The ideal speed depends :

- On the form that is being practiced
Erlu forms, for example, should always be practiced faster than Yilu forms. On the other hand, even fast forms can be practiced just quickly, or at high speed. Some forms with weapons also need more speed.

- On the student's skill
Laojia Yilu has made Taijiquan popularly known as a "slow motion" practice. This perception is in fact incorrect, as forms are practiced relatively slowly only to allow the student to develop the correct mechanics of Taijiquan movement. What does relatively slow mean? A Master can perform one round of Laojia Yilu without any quality loss in 12 to 15 minutes, which is pretty fast, but slow enough for him. Laojia Yilu usually takes 20 to 30 minutes, not more than that, except when learning choreography or in a few special cases.

- On the student's physical and aerobic capacity
Speed is limited by the student's physical fitness, the same way as in a common sport.

- On how much one has practiced that day
The first few forms in a day are always slower than in the course of that day. The body naturally warms up, gains speed and mobility within the same day. This can happen more, or less quickly, according to weather, quality of sleep the night before, and whether the student has eaten too recently or too much.

Many variables influence speed of practice. A form should not be so fast that it cannot be performed with quality, nor so slow that Qi stops circulating fluidly.

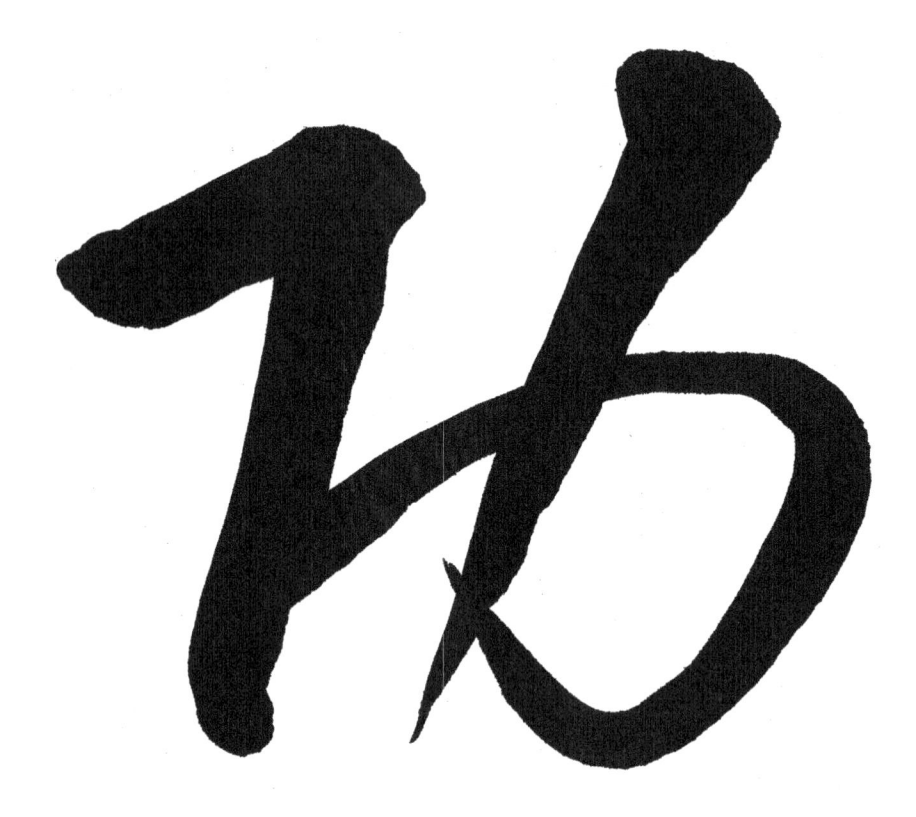

Gōngfū (功夫): work, gōng 功, beside an adult person, fū 夫. The first ideogram shows a carpenter's square, gōng 工, beside lì 力, strength: work. The second one shows a big person 大

夫

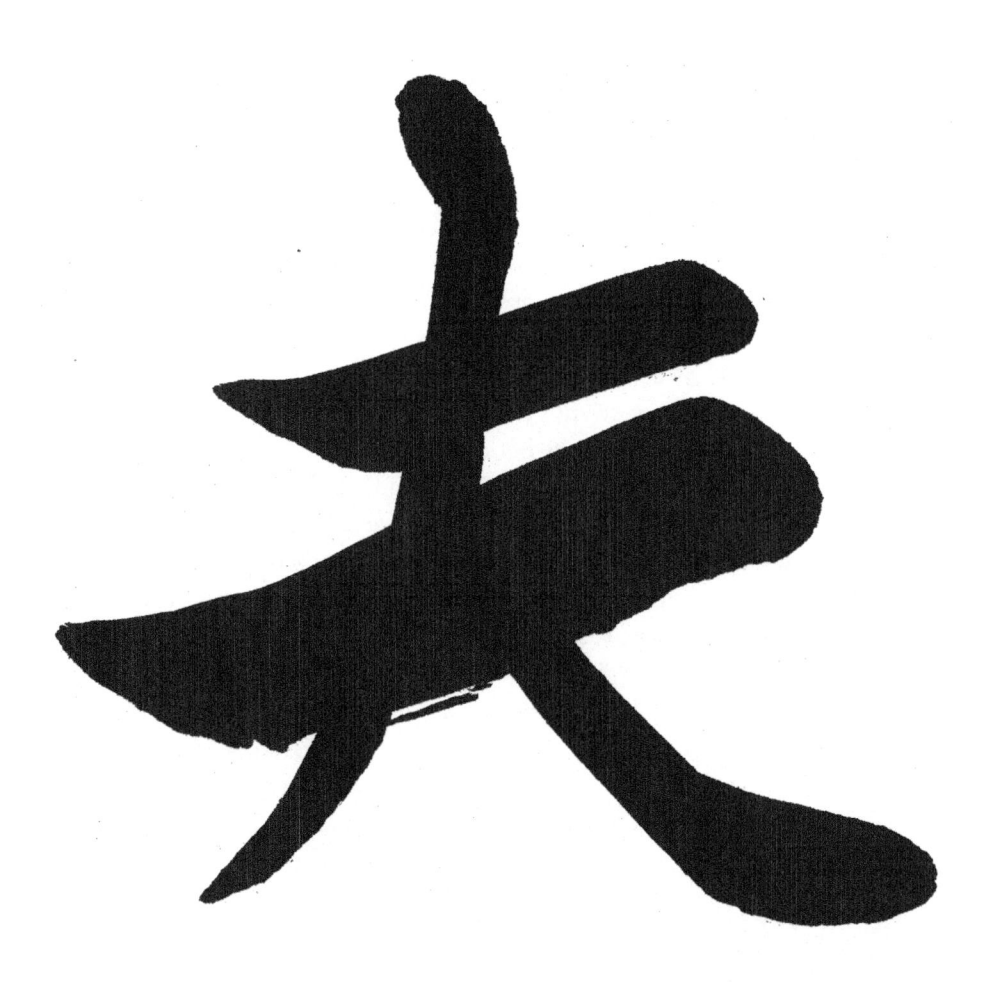

with a hairpin 一, showing the entrance into adulthood: adult, worker. Thus, a work ability that implies maturing of a skill.

Five Levels of Gongfu

In one of the occasions when I met Grandmaster Chen Xiaowang, while learning from his son Chen Yingjun in Australia, 2003, he authorized me to publish this text. Translation from Chinese to English was made by Tan Lee-Peng, Ph.D. Chen Xiaowang's essay will be regarded as a classic in future generations, since he lays a map of progress for learning Taijiquan. He does not deal with what a student would usually call technique, rather with the transformation of one's body, deepening of understanding, and increase of the student's skill. It is an extremely dense text, even tough it may not seem so at first glance. As years of practice pass, and you return to it for rereading, you will discover new meanings for the same phrases, and realize the importance of others you had not noticed before.

Chen Xiaowang mentions time estimates for completing the first through fourth levels of Gongfu. Keep in mind these estimates are not realistic at all, even for professional athletes. If you add up the estimated times, you get a prediction that it would take ten years to complete the first four levels and enter the fifth. There are probably not more than a dozen people in the world who are at the end of the third level of Gongfu. There aren't more than four or five at the fourth level. Someone beyond the middle of the third level is already regarded a Master by their peers, and if they haven't chosen seclusion, they are likely famous in Taijiquan circles. Therefore, temper expectations as you read this text, for each of the Five Levels of Gongfu is incredibly long. The introduction is much more important than you can imagine, please pay attention to it.

The text is a translation from Chinese. There are some problems in the passage from Chinese to English, which do not affect Chen Xiaowang's map of the system, but may influence the interpretation of some technical instructions. I have made small adaptations for some specific words which are usually source of confusion for western students. So, do not take the text too literally, or as a practice manual - use it for the original purpose of mapping the system.

INTRODUCTION

Learning Taijiquan is in principle similar to educating oneself, progressing from primary school to university level, while one gradually gathers more and more knowledge. Without the foundation from primary and secondary education, one will not be able to follow the courses at university level. For learning Taijiquan, one has to begin from the elementary and gradually progress to the advanced stage, level by level in a systematic manner. If one goes against this principle, thinking they could take a quick way out, they will not succeed. The whole progress of learning

Taijiquan, from the beginning to achieving success consists of five stages or five levels of martial/combat skill (Gongfu). There are objective standards for each level of Gongfu. The highest is achieved in the fifth level. The standards and martial skill requirements for each level of Gongfu will be described in the following sections. It is hoped that with these, the many Taijiquan enthusiasts all over the world will be able to assess their own current level of attainment. They will then know what they need to learn next and advance further step-by-step.

THE FIRST LEVEL OF GONGFU
In practicing Taijiquan, the requirements for different parts of the body are: keeping a straight body; keeping the head and neck erect with mindfulness at the top of the head as if one were lightly lifted by a string from above; relaxing the shoulders and sinking the elbows; relaxing the chest and waist letting them sink down; relaxing the crotch and bending the knees. When these requirements are met, one's inner energy will naturally sink down to the Dantian. Beginners may not be able to master all these important points instantly. However, in their practice, they must try to be accurate in terms of direction, angle, position, and movements of hands and legs for each posture. At this stage, one need not place too much emphasis on the requirements for different parts of the body, appropriate simplifications are acceptable. For example, for the head and upper body, it is required that the head and neck be kept erect, chest and waist be relaxed downward, but in the first level of Gongfu, it will be sufficient just to ensure that one's head and body are kept naturally upright and not leaning forward or backward, to the left or right. This is just like learning calligraphy, at the beginning, one needs only to make sure that the strokes are correct. Therefore, when practicing Taijiquan at the beginning, the body and movements may appear to be stiff; or "externally solid but internally empty". One may find oneself doing things like: hard hitting, ramming, sudden uplifting and/or sudden collapsing of body or trunk. There may also be broken or over-exerted force or Jin. All these faults are common to beginners. If one is persistent enough and practices seriously everyday, one can normally know the forms within half a year. The inner energy, Qi, can gradually be induced to move within the trunk and limbs with refinements in one's movements. One may then achieve the stage of "being able to use external movements to channel internal energy". The first level Gongfu thus begins with knowing the postures to gradually being able to detect and understand Jin or force.

The martial skill attainable with the first level of Gongfu is very limited. This is because at this stage, one's actions are not well coordinated and systematic. The postures may not be correct. Thus the force or Jin that is produced may be stiff, broken, lax, or on the other hand too strong. When practicing the routine, one's postures may appear hollow or angular. As such one can only feel the internal energy but is not able to channel the energy to every part of the body in one go. Consequently, one is not able to harness the force or Jin right from the heels, channel it up the legs, and discharge it through command of the centre. On the contrary, beginners can only produce broken force that "surges" from one section to another section of the body. Therefore the first level Gongfu is insufficient for martial application purposes. If one were to test one's skill on someone who does not know martial arts, they can remain flexible to a certain extent. They may not have mastered the application but by knowing how to mislead their opponent the student may occasionally be able to throw them off. Even then, they may be unable to maintain their own balance. Such a situation is thus termed "10% Yin and 90% Yang; top-heavy staff".

What then exactly is Yin and Yang? In the context of practicing Taijiquan, emptiness is Yin, solidity is Yang; gentleness or softness is Yin, forcefulness or hardness is Yang. Yin-Yang is the unity of the opposites; neither one cannot be left out; yet both can be mutually interchanged and transformed. If we assign a maximum of 100% to measure them, when one in their practice can attain an equal balance of Yin and Yang, they are said to have achieved 50% Yin and 50% Yang. This is the highest standard or an indication of success in practicing Taijiquan. In the first level of skill or Gongfu, it is normal for one to end up with "10% Yin and 90% Yang". That is, one's Quan or boxing is more hard than soft and there is imbalance in Yin and Yang. The student is not able to complement hard with soft and to command applications with ease. As such, while still at the first level, students should not be too eager to pursue the application aspect in each posture.

THE SECOND LEVEL OF GONGFU
The level starting from the last stage of the first level, when one can feel the movement of internal energy or Qi, to the early stage of the third level of Gongfu is termed as the second level of Gongfu. The second level of Gongfu involves further reducing shortcomings such as: stiff force or Jin produced while practicing Taijiquan; over- and under-exertion of force as well as movements which are not well coordinated. This is to ensure that the internal energy (Qi) will move systematically in the body in accordance with the requirements of each movement. Eventually, this should result in smooth flowing of Qi in the body and good coordination of internal Qi with external movements.

After acquiring the first level of Gongfu, one should be able to practice with ease according to the preliminary requirements of the movements. The student is able to feel the movement of internal energy. However, the student may not be able to control the flow of Qi in the body. There are two reasons for this: firstly, the student has not accurately mastered the specific requirements on each part of the body and their coordination. As an example, if the chest is relaxed downward too much, the hips and back may not be straight, or if the hips are too relaxed then the chest and rear may protrude. As such, one must further strictly ensure that the requirements on each part of the body should be resolved so that they move in unison. This will enable the whole body to unite in a coordinated manner (which means coordinated internal and external harmonies. Internal harmonies implies coordinated union of heart and mind, of internal energy and force, tendons and bones. External harmonies implies coordinated union of hands with feet, elbows with knees, shoulders with hips). Simultaneously, there should be an equal and opposite closing movement of another part of the body and vice versa. Opening and closing movements come together and complement each other. Secondly, while practicing one may find it hard to control different parts of the body all at once. This means one part of the body may move faster than the rest and result in over-exertion of force; or a certain part may move too slowly or without enough force, thus resulting in an under-exertion of force. These two phenomena both contradict the principle of Taijiquan. Every movement in Chen style Taijiquan is required not to deviate from the principle of the "spiralling-silk force" or Chansijin. According to the theory of Taijiquan, "'Chansijin originates from the kidneys and is found at all times in every part of the body". In the process of learning Taijiquan, the spiralling-silk method of movement (ie. the twining and spiralling method of movement) and the spiralling-silk force (ie. the inner force produced from the spiralling-silk method of movement), can be strictly mastered through relaxing shoulders and elbows, chest and hips as well as crotch and knees and using the centre as a pivot to move every part of the body. Starting with rotating the hands inward, the hands should lead the elbows which in turn lead the shoulders which then guide the centre (the part of the centre corresponding to that side of the shoulder that is being moved. In actual fact the centre is still the pivot). On the other hand, if the hands rotate in an outward direction, the centre should move the shoulders, the shoulders move the elbows, the elbows in turn move the hands. For the upper half of the body, the wrists and arms should appear to be gyrating; whereas for the lower portion of the body the ankles and the thighs should appear to be rotating; as for the trunk, the hips and the back should appear to be turning. Combining the movements of the three parts of the body we should visualize a curve rotating in space. This curve originates from the legs, with the centre at the hips and ends at the fingers. In practicing the Quan (the form), if one feels awkward with a particular movement, one can adjust one's hips and thighs according to the sequence of flow of Chansijin to achieve coordination. In this way, any error can be corrected. Therefore, while paying attention to the requirements for each part of the body to achieve total coordination of the whole body, the mastering of the rhythm of movement of the spiralling silk method and spiralling silk force is a way of resolving conflicts and self-correction for any mistake in practicing Taijiquan after attaining the second level of Gongfu.

In the first level of Gongfu, one begins with learning the forms, and when one is familiar with the forms, they can feel the movement of internal energy in the body. The student may well be very excited and thus never feel tired or bored. However, in entering the second level of Gongfu, the student may feel there is nothing new to learn and at the same time misunderstand certain important points. The student may not have mastered these main points accurately and thus find that their movements are awkward. Or, on the other hand, the student may find that they can practice the Quan smoothly and express force with much vigour but cannot apply them while doing push-hands. Because of this, one may soon feel bored, lose confidence and may give up altogether. The only way to reach the stage where one can: produce the right amount of force, not too hard and not too soft; change actions at will; and turn smoothly with ease, is to be persistent and strictly adhere to principles. One has to train hard in the form so that the body movements are well coordinated, and with "one single movement can activate movements in every part of the body", thus establishing a complete system of movements. There is a common saying, "if the principle is not clearly understood, consult with a teacher; if the way is not clearly visible, seek the help of friends". When the principles as well as the methods are clearly understood, with constant practice, success will eventually prevail. The Taijiquan Classics state that, "everybody can possess the ultimate, if only one works hard." And "if only one persists, ultimately one should achieve sudden breakthrough". Generally, most people can attain the second level of Gongfu in about four years. When one reaches the state of being able to experience a smooth flow of Qi in the body, one would suddenly understand it (the command of Qi) all. When this happens, one will be full of confidence and enthusiasm as one goes on practicing. One may even have the strong urge to go on and on and won't feel like stopping!

At the beginning of the second level of Gongfu the martial art skill attained is about the same as in the first level Gongfu. It is not sufficient for actual application. At the end of the second level Gongfu one is nearly entering the third level of Gongfu, as such the martial skill acquired may be applicable to a certain extent.

The next section introduces the martial skill that should be attainable half-way through the second level of Gongfu (so are the third, fourth and fifth levels of Gongfu in the subsequent sections. They are discussed with reference to the skill attainable in the half-way stage in each level.)

Push-hands and practicing Taijiquan are inseparable. Whatever shortcomings one has in their Quan (form) will show up as weaknesses during push-hands thus giving the opponent an opportunity to take advantage of them. Because of this, in practicing Taijiquan every part of one's body must be well coordinated with the rest, there shouldn't be any unnecessary movements. Push-hands requires warding-off, grabbing, squeezing and pressing (Peng, Lu, Ji, An) to be carried out so precisely that the upper and lower parts of the body move in coordination and it is thus difficult for opponents to attack. As the saying goes: "No matter how great is the force on me, I should mobilize four ounces of strength to deflect one thousand pounds of force". The second level of Gongfu aims at achieving smooth flowing of Qi in the body by correcting the postures so as to reach the stage where Qi should penetrate the whole body passing through every joint as if it (Qi) is sequentially linked. However, the process of adjusting the postures involves making unnecessary or uncoordinated movements. Therefore, at this stage, one is unable to apply the martial skill at will during push-hands. The opponent will concentrate on looking for these weaknesses or they may win by surprising one in committing errors like over-exerting, collapsing, throwing-off and confronting of force. During push-hands, the opponent's advance will not allow one to have time to adjust one's movements. The opponent will make use of one's weak point to attack so that one will lose balance or will be forced to step back to ward off the advancing force. Nevertheless, if the opponent advances with less force and in a slower manner, there may be time or opportunity to make adjustments and one may be able to ward off the attack in a more satisfactory manner. Drawing from the above discussion, for the second level of Gongfu, whether one is attacking or blocking-off an attack, much effort is needed. Very often, it will be an advantage to make the first move, the one who moves last will be at a disadvantage. At this level, one is unable to "forget oneself and play along with the opponent" (i.e. not to attack but to yield to the opponent's movement); unable to grasp an opportunity to respond to change. One may be able to move and ward off an attack but may easily commit errors like throwing-off or collapsing and over-exerting or confronting force. Because of these errors, during push-hands, one cannot move according to the sequence of warding-off, grabbing, squeezing and pressing. A person with this level of skill is described as "20% Yin, 80% Yang: an undisciplined new hand."

THE THIRD LEVEL OF GONGFU

"If you wish to do well in your Quan (form), you must practice to make your circles smaller." The steps in practicing Chen style Taijiquan involve progressing from mastering big circles to medium circles and from medium circles to small circles. The word "circle" here does not mean the path resulting from the movements of the limbs, rather the smooth flow of the internal energy (Qi). In this respect, the third level of Gongfu is a stage in which one shall begin with big circles and end with medium circles (in the circulation of Qi).

The Taijiquan Classic mentions that "Yi and Qi are superior to forms", meaning that while practicing Taijiquan one should place emphasis on using Yi (consciousness). In the first level of Gongfu, one's mind and concentration are mainly on learning and mastering the external forms of Taijiquan. While in the second level of Gongfu, one should concentrate on detecting conflicts and un-coordination of limbs and body and of internal energy and external movements. One should adjust body and forms to ensure a smooth flow of internal energy. When progressing into the third level of Gongfu, one should already have the internal energy flowing smoothly: what is required is Qi and not brute force. The movements should be light but not "floating", heavy but not clumsy. This implies that the movements should appear to be soft but the internal force is actually strong, sturdy, or there is strong force implied in the soft movements, and the whole body should be well coordinated and there should not be any irregular movements. However, one should not just pay attention to the movement of Qi in the body and neglect the external actions. Otherwise, one would appear to be in a daze, and as a result the flow of internal Qi might not only be obstructed but dispersed. Therefore, as stated in the Taijiquan Classic, "attention should be on the spirit and not just Qi, with too much emphasis on Qi, there will be stagnation (of Qi)."

One may have mastered the external forms between the first and second levels of Gongfu, but they may not have attained coordination of the external movements with the internal. Sometimes, due to stiffness or stagnation of the actions, full breathing in is not possible. On the other hand, without proper coordination of the internal and external movements, it is not possible to empty one's breath completely. Thus when practicing Quan one should breath naturally. After entering the third level of Gongfu, there is better coordination of internal and external movements, as such, generally the actions can be synchronized with breathing quite precisely. However, it is necessary to consciously synchronize breathing with movements for some finer, more complicated and swifter actions. This is to further ensure coordination of breathing and actions so that it gradually comes on naturally.

The third level of Gongfu basically involves mastering the internal and external requirements of Chen style Taijiquan and rhythm of exercise, as well as the ability to correct oneself. One should also be able to command the actions with more ease and should also have more internal energy (Qi). At this level, it is necessary to further understand the combat skill implicit in each posture and its applications. For this, one has to practice push hands, and check in the forms the quality and quantity of the internal force and expression of the force as well as the dissolving of the force. If one's postures can withstand confrontational push hands then one must have mastered the important points of the form. They would gain more confidence if they continue to work hard. They may then step up their exercise routine and add in some complementary practices such as long staff, sword or broadsword, spear and staff as well as practicing Fajin (expression of explosive force) on its own. With two years of continuous practice in this manner, generally one should be able to attain the fourth level of Gongfu.

With the third level of Gongfu, although there is smooth flow of internal Qi and the actions are better coordinated, internal Qi is still too weak and coordination between muscle movements and the functioning of the internal organs is not sufficiently established. While practicing alone without external disturbances one may be able to achieve internal and external coordination. During confrontational push hands and combat, if the advancing force is softer and slower, one may be able to go along with the attacker and change one's actions accordingly, grab any opportunity to lead the opponent in a disadvantageous situation, or avoid the opponent's firm move but attack when there is any weakness, maneuvering with ease. However, once encountering a stronger opponent, the student may feel that their Pengjin is insufficient, and there is a feeling that one's posture is being pressed and about to collapse (this may destroy the unfailing position which is supposed to be never-leaning and never-declining but with all around support), and cannot maneuver at will. The student may not achieve what the Taijiquan Classic describes as "striking with the hands without them being seen, once they are visible, it is impossible to manipulate". Even in leading-in and expelling-out the opponent, one may feel stiff and much effort is required. As such, the skill at this stage is described as "30% Yin, 70% Yang, still on the hard side".

THE FOURTH LEVEL OF GONGFU
Progressing from the stage with medium circles to that with small circles is required at the fourth level of Gongfu. This is the stage nearing success and thus is of high level of Gongfu. One should have mastered the effective method of training, be able to grasp the important points

in the movements, be able to understand the martial/combat skill implicit in each movement, have smooth flow of the internal energy (Qi), and have coordination of actions and breathing. However, during practice, each step and each movement of hands should be carried out with a confronting opponent in mind, that is to say, one has to assume that they are surrounded by enemies. For each posture and each form, each part of the body must move in a linked and continuous manner so that the whole body moves in unison. "Movements of the upper and lower body are related and there should be a continuous flow of Qi with the control being at the centre" so that when practicing forms, one should carry it out "as if there is an opponent although no one is around". When actually confronted, one should be brave but cautious, behaving "as if there is no one around though there is someone there."

The training content (like empty-hand forms and weapons) is similar to that in third level of Gongfu. With perseverance, generally the fifth level Gongfu can be reached in three years. In terms of martial skill the fourth level differs much from the third level Gongfu. The third level Gongfu aims at dissolving the opponent's force and getting rid of conflicts in one's own actions. This is to enable one to play the active role and forcing the opponent to be passive. The fourth level of Gongfu enables one to dissolve as well as express force. This is because at that level, one would have sufficient internal Jin, flexible change in Yi and Qi and a consolidated system of the body movements. As such, during push-hands, the opponent's attack does not pose a big threat. On contact with the opponent, one can immediately change one's action and thus dissolve the oncoming force with ease, exhibiting the special characteristics of going along with the movements of the opponent yet changing one's own actions all the time to counteract the opponent's action, exerting the right force, adjusting internally, predicting the opponent's intention, subduing one's own actions, expressing precise force and hitting the target accurately. Therefore, a person attaining this level of Gongfu is described as "40% Yin, 60% Yang; akin to a good practitioner."

THE FIFTH LEVEL OF GONGFU

The fifth level Gongfu is the stage in which one progresses from commanding small circles to commanding invisible circles, from mastering the form to executing the form invisibly. According to the Taijiquan Classics, "with the continuous smooth flowing of Qi, with the cosmic Qi moving one's natural internal Qi, moving from a fixed form to invisibility, one realizes how wonderful nature is." At the fifth level, actions should be flexible and smooth, and there should be sufficient internal Jin. However, it is still necessary to strive for the best. There is a need to work hard day by day until the body is very flexible and adaptable to multi-faceted changes. There should be changes internally alternating between the substantial and insubstantial but these should be invisible externally. Only then the fifth level of Gongfu is achieved.

Regarding martial skill, at this level the gang (hard) should complement the rou (soft), the form should be relaxed, dynamic, springy and lively. Every move and every motionless instant is in accordance with the Taiji principle, as are the movements of the whole body. This means that every part of the body should be very sensitive and quick to react when the need arises. So much so that every part of the body can act as a fist to attack whenever it is in contact with the opponent's body. There should also be constant interchange between expressing and conserving of force and the posture should be firm as though supported from all sides.

Therefore the description for this level of Gongfu is "only one that moves with 50% Yin and 50% Yang, without any bias towards Yin or Yang, is termed a good master. A good master makes every move according to the Taiji principles which demand every move be invisible."

After completing the fifth level of Gongfu a strong relationship has been established between the coordination of the mind, contraction and relaxation of the muscles, movements of the muscles and functioning of the internal organs. Even when encountering a sudden attack such coordination will not be hampered as one should be flexible to change. Even then, one should continue to pursue further so as to achieve greater heights.

Development in science is without boundaries, so is practicing Taijiquan: one could never exhaust all its beauty and benefits in one's life time.

Further reading

We suggest following the author's website, https://taijiquan-ottawa.com, which is updated regularly. Links can be found there to his social media profiles, good books on Taijiquan, and videos of the Masters.

VIDEOS

There is an almost inexhaustible amount of material available on Youtube. It's okay to watch demonstrations from various sources, but it's important for your learning that when you're studying — that is, analyzing movement, or following the video — your choice be Grandmaster Chen Xiaowang. There is no better source. Following other teachers may seem tempting because of their movements' beauty or dexterity, but it's easy to find videos that introduce small defects in movement that you don't consciously notice, or videos that, while technically correct, may not be most productive from a didactic point of view.

BOOKS

The author is presently writing a sequel to this volume.

You should read any and everything Grandmaster Chen Xiaowang has written. Likewise, we advise you acquire the books by Master Jan Silberstorff, who besides being a Taijiquan Master at a high technical level, is a very prolific author and has very clear didactics. David Gaffney and Davidine von Sim are also authors we recommend for their technical solidity, whose books will contribute to your learning.

Chen Xin, the most prominent Master in the 16th generation of the Chen Family, wrote a treatise called Chenshi Taijiquan Tushuo. This treatise is used to this day by Masters in the Chen family to study the technical details of their art. I have been told that understanding it would only be possible when I no longer needed to read it. When I met Chen Xiaowang during his second seminar in Brazil, I asked him if I could try and find a translator for the book, as at that time he had not yet published any Western-language works. He replied that it would not be worth it to undertake a translation that would not be done by an expert in Taijiquan, as every sentence of that treatise was like a book in itself. All images from Chapter 2, and images 3.9.1, and 3.9.6 to 3.9.8 are part of Chen Xin's Taijiquan Tushuo.

This book was composed in Chaparral Pro 11/13.2 pt.
Originally, pollen paper 80 g/m2 was used.

Its composition took place throughout the 2020 pandemic. In such a dramatic moment when so many perished, it was a joy bringing to light a work dedicated to Taijiquan, a pearl from Chinese civilization.

As wise advice in hexagram 36 of the I Ching, translated by Richard Wilhelm, reminds us:

"Dimming of the light. It is favourable to persevere during adversity."

Printed in Great Britain
by Amazon